My Story to Yours

MY STORY TO YOURS

A Guided Memoir for Writing
Your Recovery Journey

ॐ

Karen Casey, Ph.D.

HAZELDEN

Hazelden
Center City, Minnesota 55012
hazelden.org

Library of Congress Cataloging-in-Publication Data
Casey, Karen.
     My story to yours : a guided memoir for writing your recovery
journey / Karen Casey.
          p. cm.
     ISBN 978-1-61649-094-2 (softcover)—ISBN 978-1-61649-163-5
(e-book)
     1. Alcoholics—Rehabilitation. 2. Autobiography—Therapeutic use.
3. Diaries—Authorship—Therapeutic use. 4. Casey, Karen. I.Title.
     HV5275.C373 2011
     362.292092—dc23
     [B]

                                                          2011020014

Editor's note

Some names, details, and circumstances have been changed to
protect the privacy of those mentioned in this publication.

This publication is not intended as a substitute for the advice
of health care professionals.

Alcoholics Anonymous and AA are registered trademarks of
Alcoholics Anonymous World Services, Inc.

15   14   13   2   3   4   5   6

Cover design by David Spohn
Interior design and typesetting by Percolator Graphic Design

As has been true in many other books, I dedicate this one to my husband, Joe. He has been in my corner since the late 1970s, giving me words of encouragement when I need them and reasons to laugh when I need those too. He is the companion I always dreamed of having.

CONTENTS

ACKNOWLEDGMENTS

I WANT TO THANK HAZELDEN, particularly Sid Farrar, for once again being a champion for my work. I have been comfortably in their care for many decades now and hope our relationship continues. I want to acknowledge my many friends inside and outside of the recovery rooms. Without their wisdom and constant presence, my journey would be far less peaceful. And then there's my Higher Power, without whom I'd still be trying to figure out who I am and what my work is supposed to be. How very grateful I am every day of my life.

WRITING HAS BEEN my emotional and spiritual life-line for decades. In my youth, I wrote long, tedious, and dramatic stories describing in detail a family of origin that I wished had been mine—one very different from my argumentative and emotionally distant family. Throughout grade school and high school, I continued to long for this other, very loving, very present family. My longing prevented me from appreciating, from even noticing, the lessons that were available to me in my real family—lessons that I came to realize had been selected especially for me.

In graduate school, writing continued to sustain me emotionally. In fact, it became a transformative experience, which was something I had certainly not expected. Regardless of the college course I was taking or the topic I was researching, I tackled the many papers I had to write with an unexpected ease. I looked forward to them, in fact. The accumulation of A's astounded me, and the year I spent writing a 300-page dissertation offered me a daily, natural high.

My friends were envious, for sure. And frankly, I was stunned by my experience. I knew I was no scholar, not on the level of most others in my classes. I think there is an explanation for my ease of writing, however—one that I will share in a later section of the book. For now, let me just say that when God has a plan, nothing stands in the way as long as we have even the slightest bit of willingness.

In 1980, in the midst of great personal emotional turmoil and overriding fear, the meditations that were to become *Each Day a New Beginning,* my first published book, tumbled forth as though I were having a conversation with God. The same has been true of every book I've written since then. I sit quietly and the words and the ideas form unbidden in my mind. My willingness to write them down is my part of the equation.

When it was time for me to start writing this memoir, though, an unexpected and unfamiliar feeling emerged. I felt blocked. I was almost afraid to begin. It was, I believe, more subtle than the writer's block so many writers complain about, but I couldn't break the spell. I sensed a shadow enveloping me, a shadow not unlike the one I had lived with for so many years before and during early recovery. I woke up with the shadow. I went to bed with it. It followed me everywhere. It gripped my mind for many days. I could feel a fear creeping into my psyche. I feared that this shadow was to be my new persona. And I was filled with an awful dread.

I didn't stay under the covers, although I surely wanted to. In a blur I went about my days much as I always had— my daily workouts, meetings, commitments with friends— but I was going through the motions rather than living the experiences. My patience wore thin at the grocery store, in traffic, even in meetings. And I was more than a little edgy with my husband. Most of all, I felt impatient with my stuck state of mind.

I have been in recovery from the effects of alcohol and drug addiction since 1974. In recovery, my nature has always been to welcome people who come into "my space." But now these people felt like intruders. The invisibility I had felt for so many years before coming into recovery was nipping at the edges of my mind. I hated how I was feeling and acting, but I couldn't shake it off. Or perhaps *wouldn't* shake it off. I wasn't sure. It felt as if I were in the throes of an emotional tantrum. The ease with which my friends laughed, and my husband too, heightened how separate I felt from all of them.

Before getting up each morning, I tried to sense my emotional state. Would today be the day I felt like me again? And then I did a lead at a meeting, one I had signed up to do a few weeks earlier when life had looked far cheerier. Not knowing what I was going to say, I simply opened my mouth and began talking about the shadow—how the darkness felt, what the fear had done to me, how I had reverted to the person I had been so many years before. I told the group how withdrawn I'd become and how my favorite gatherings were no longer enjoyable. I didn't feel like me. I explained that I didn't like the person that I feared I had become and that I was devastated by my regression.

As I talked, a light shone on my shadow, and it ever so slightly began to lift. I had talked about it to my husband and a few close friends, but not in detail, and my superficial remarks had changed nothing. It was as though I chose to suffer in silence. And I felt ashamed. After all, I had three and a half decades of recovery. I led workshops, wrote books, and gave lectures. How could I be stuck in this emotional quagmire?

In hindsight, I firmly believe that for most of my professional, *and recovery* life, I had made an investment in having others see me "in a better light," without even being conscious of it. But on that day, I told the group exactly who I was in that very moment.

With each new revelation, I could see more clearly. I could see how I had created a wall around me that only I could dismantle. As the group listened attentively, and as I took in their expressions of love, I felt an ease that had not been present for some time. I could even sense my breathing change. My shoulders, so often tense, relaxed once again. And the many, ever-so-helpful principles I had learned in Twelve Step meetings that until recently had been my safety net, came rushing back. *Let go, just let go,* rang in my ears.

My relief was palpable. God had begun to do for me what my worry had not accomplished. Worry never serves us. Once again I needed reminding that I had edged God out and, as a result, whatever I focused on got bigger, both the good and the bad. I needed reminding that until I truly turned everything over to the God of my understanding, He couldn't unravel any confusion or heighten any joy I might feel.

As I closed the meeting, I looked around the circle of

men and women. I saw them differently in that moment, and I could feel the change deep within me. They had a softness about them, a gentleness in their smiles, an acceptance in their nods toward me. They understood my words. I had spoken their truth too. And the wall existed no more.

I tell this story because I want to stress how the journey we are traveling is seldom free from unexpected curves or unnecessary walls. Writing one's life story is important because it gives us a chance to sit back and take the long view of our lives, noting in the process the tiny details that are so easily passed over when telling one's story. Because this memoir is intended to help both me and you as a reader and writer reclaim all of who we were and are now, writing helps to establish the flow for easier access into the recesses of one's mind. I'm of the opinion that we can't actually move forward successfully if we aren't willing to see where we have been. The good news is that it's on the curves and behind the walls that we get our opportunities for growth, those opportunities that we were born to experience. Speaking our truth is what heals us and others too. The telling of our stories, coupled with the writing of them, offers both us and the "witness" to our story a depth that is often lost if we limit our sharing of it to "the stage." We need to delve deep into the recesses of our minds, which can seldom be accomplished in the kind of setting where we simply speak. Our paths cross because our truths need to intersect and inform one another. What a glorious awareness this is—one that can be forgotten but also reclaimed. I'd like to say that I'll construct no more walls, but that would no doubt be a lie. My humanity, my fear, has a pile of bricks in the wings. But my heart will always find a way to dismantle it. That is the most important truth of all.

M Y NAME IS KAREN, and I'm an alcoholic. But I am more than that label and that's what I will explore in the pages of this book. Labels limit us, even though they also help define us. Was I always an alcoholic? Was that first drink at thirteen, poured before the unseeing eyes of my parents, the event that determined the rest of my journey? Or have the many other experiences through many decades of living contributed equally to the woman who sits here now scouring the past to share what it was like, what happened, and the glory of what it's like now?

When I began considering a memoir as my next book, I knew I wanted to do something different from myriad other memoirs in the bookstores. It's not that the lives of others aren't interesting. On the contrary, reading the behind-the-scenes moments of the semiprivate lives of famous and not-so-famous folks is seductive. But I wanted you to want to read this book because it was different from the many others that may have called to you in the past.

Let me be clear: my story is not spectacular. Many women have stories far more explosive or glamorous than mine. My story is quite ordinary, in fact. But I wanted to do more than ask you to read my story; I wanted to interest you in exploring your own story, along with me, within the context of specific suggestions, as well as within the ever-so-common format of what it was like, what happened, and what it's like now. I base the writing prompts, the questions for you to explore and write about, on memories that stood out for me, memories that seemed to cover the many ways I had changed in the thirty-seven years (as of this writing) since I walked into my first recovery meeting. I'm hoping the questions will resonate with you too. And if they don't, perhaps they will at least prompt a memory that will excite you as you explore, with the help of this guide, your own journey from then until now.

We are changed by our experiences, each one of them. Every person we have contact with makes his indelible mark too. And every event leaves traces of our having "been there" in our minds and in the minds of those with whom we shared those moments. The details may live in the shadows for years, but live they do. It's into those shadows that I go in the pages that follow. What I discovered are parts of myself that I had skirted in the many years that have passed since I lived the experiences.

There is no single correct way to write your own memoir. And doing it in longhand will appeal to some who think the computer makes them once-removed from the life they are sharing. Personally, I think using the computer improves my flow in sharing what I want to say. I can type faster and with less physical pain than writing in longhand. Personal preference is the key, however.

When you choose to write will depend on personal preference too. If you are moved to share instantly because of the fear that a particular thought will be lost if you do not write it down immediately, then by all means, write it down. Many of you will choose to read the entire book, as an inspiration of sorts, before delving into your own story. Again, let me reiterate, there is no one way or right way to do this. The process of doing it is what's important.

The excitement I feel for my discoveries is appreciable. Sharing my discoveries with you doubles the pleasure. It's my hope, and the underlying intention of this book, that you will grow in awareness of the details of your own journey—of your countless successes, as well as your opportunities for continued growth. I hope you will feel at the end of this shared experience that you have moved into being more of the person your Higher Power has always known you'd be.

Because the details of my life will emerge as we move forward together, I prefer to limit my personal remarks for now. But, rest assured, I was careening out of control before someone suggested those fateful words to me in 1974: "I think you should go to Al-Anon." I was a fear-filled third child in a rage-filled family of four children for more than three decades before finally hearing those words. And I didn't rest securely in the information I heard at the meetings I was regularly attending until the repetition penetrated my stubborn resistance. When the student is ready, the teacher does appear.

It's my hope to serve, in some capacity, as the teacher

on your path at this very moment. My guess is that's the reason you chose this book at this very moment. Looking together at who we have been, who we are now, and how we got here is a gift we deserve to open and cherish. If not now, when? Let's take the journey together, shall we?

Revisiting Our Journeys—Together

"Hi, Toyce, it's me. Is it morning or night?"

"What's happened to you, Karen? Are you okay?"

"Nothing has happened; I'm fine," I said, laughing. "I'm just wondering if it's time to go to bed or time to get ready for our class."

"It's evening. Don't you remember that we celebrated your birthday last night and then went our separate ways about 10 p.m.?"

"I guess not. Sure am glad it's time to go to bed though. See you tomorrow."

And from that moment on, nothing was ever the same.

S IFTING THROUGH THE MEMORIES of one's childhood can be exciting as well as traumatic. My excitement while exploring the themes for this book has been in recalling many good times that I had with my family and friends (fortunately, I did not forget them all completely). Like many people, I lived in the bad memories for too much of my life. Good memories are always intertwined with the bad, but some of us more easily hang on to those memories that troubled us out of fear of who we'd be if we let them go. Perhaps their indelible markings seem more prominent, and they serve as great excuses for our lack of success in many avenues of our life.

I have tried to be open to all the stories behind the many images from my past that come to mind, some of them triggered by photos I still possess. Some memories triggered a quick smile. Some made me laugh out loud. Good memories are worth savoring always, but at this time in my life, they are extremely significant. Good memories can change everything about the life we recall if we give them a place of honor in our minds. I have made a commitment to do just that. Perhaps you'll join me.

Make a note to yourself, right now, to search for the photos from your youth to dwell on as fodder for the story you need to tell about yourself. This is a great exercise, and one that you can share with a loved one too.

I intend to highlight those good memories, weaving them into the tapestry that is me, not only because of the freedom they offer me now, but because fond memories help our hearts heal—a belief that has been proven scientifically.

Now I invite you to think about those experiences from your life that make you smile, along with those that you've cried over, as you wander with me through some of my life's experiences. You may be inclined to journal about some of your memories as we travel this path together—at least that's my hope for you. So get a notebook and pen to have handy. You'll need them. Initiating my exploration beneath the surface has been a blessing to me. And I trust that you will be grateful for your discoveries too.

Have your notebook or journal and your pen or pencil by you as you read this memoir. If you find you are being drawn into too many of your memories all at once, jot down a note or two about each memory, enough to trigger a full recall later when you have more time to write. That's an exercise I have used for years and it works wonderfully well.

What It Was Like

࿎

EARLY PATHS I FOLLOWED

THE 1940s, the decade of my childhood, seems so long ago. Today I sit in a comfortable home on a lake in Minnesota, just south of the Twin Cities, amazed that this is the journey my Higher Power selected for me. I am generally confident, certain that my journey will continue to carry me into the experiences that will bless and stretch me at the same time. And I no longer doubt that who I am meeting and what I am asked to do are the next right invitations for me to experience. But none of this was the case prior to 1974. None of it.

In my childhood, as the third in my family of four children, I vacillated between two extremes: feelings of overwhelming uncertainty and overbearing boldness. The boldness was a cover-up for fear, no doubt, a reaction to my dad, who seemed to bully my mom and my younger brother. I proudly stood my ground with him, and tried to stand their ground too. It gained us nothing. My mother wasn't helped by my aggression. Nor was my brother. And I felt disempowered and chastened again and again.

WHAT IT WAS LIKE

My father wasn't a bad man. On the contrary. He was a
respected member of our 30,000-member community and
held an important position at the largest bank in town. He
was simply a scared man. A very scared man. Fear ruled
his life. Fear is insidious and contagious. It can permeate a
family. It certainly permeated ours. I came to understand
the depth of his fear early in my own recovery, a story I will
share later in this memoir. But I want it to be known that
he did not abuse anyone physically or sexually, although a
spanking wasn't out of the question. He expressed his fear
by yelling and swearing—a lot. And his raised voice, which
the neighbors could hear, scared me and humiliated my
mom on a regular basis. The tears sliding down her face
are etched in my memory to this day.

One experience that left its mark on my mind happened
when I was eight or nine. It was Friday evening and we
were having supper, my three siblings, my parents, and I.
Hamburgers were our standard fare on Fridays. I'll never
know what triggered my dad's behavior that night, but he
sat in his usual place, directly across from my mother at
our small kitchen table, and he lined up the ketchup bottle
just so. It had the kind of dispenser that you tapped on
and the ketchup dripped out. After aiming the bottle just
right, he made a fist and came down hard on top of the
dispenser. You can envision what came next. Ketchup flew
across the table and splattered my mother squarely in the
face. Her glasses protected her eyes, but nothing protected
her against the humiliation. With tears streaming down

her face and mixing with the ketchup, she headed to the bathroom and didn't return to the table. My father offered us her unfinished hamburger, but I could barely finish my own because of my nausea over what had just occurred.

We sat in stunned silence at first. Then I remember, as though it were yesterday, my dad had a strangely satisfied look on his face. My older sisters laughed nervously, but my brother Jim and I were quiet. We didn't look at dad or anyone. Perhaps we feared this was the beginning of the end of our family. I don't know, but I do remember that my parents rarely spoke in the evenings after that. They read the evening paper and listened to the radio or, after 1952, watched television. Following the ten o'clock news, my parents called it a day.

As a middle child, I swung among the roles of hopeful peacemaker; silent, anxious observer; and protector of my mom and younger brother. My father was angry much of the time. Depressed, perhaps, but unmedicated. He seethed below the surface some days and verbally raged on many others. You could sense his mood even upon rising in the mornings and certainly the minute he entered the kitchen following work. What I didn't know as a child was that he was as afraid as I was most of the time. Because of his fear that he wasn't perfect, he projected his need for perfection on all of us. Naturally we fell short. On a daily basis we fell short—as did he.

One summer day I fell short in front of my best friend. Someone had tracked dirt into the house, and the evidence was on the hardwood floor between the living and dining rooms. My dad, who was home that day because of a migraine headache, asked me to clean it up, and following my ten-year-old mind, I went to the kitchen and got the broom and dustpan. This incensed my dad. He had expected me to get the vacuum, which had never occurred to me. He rose from his chair, grabbed me, turned me over his knee, pulled down my pants, and spanked me. In front of Barbara. I was mortified—and furious and adamant that I would not shed a tear. Barbara and I retreated upstairs, and I pretended the spanking didn't hurt. I silently vowed to pay him back, and I would get my chance.

At the time of this incident, I wish I had known more about fear and its capacity to immobilize us. I would learn later in life that my father lived with a lot of emotional pain. That he became a successful banker, looked up to by the community, was owing to his undying need to be more than he ever felt he really was. And I followed in his footsteps. He taught me well.

When I went into my dad's bank, people treated me with respect too, because I was his daughter, and I felt proud. I knew a very different man at home, but I was glad his employees looked up to him. I wanted their respect for him to change the man we saw at home, but that wasn't to be, at least not on a typical day. I have come to cherish the wise words of the "elders" I first encountered in the rooms of AA and Al-Anon: "Our parents did the best they could." These words didn't lessen all the pain I struggled to understand from my own life, but they did help me to see a different father—the man behind the words and actions.

YOUR TIME TO WRITE: Recalling how the good and the bad situations in our past provide a balance that continues to inform us, a balance that promises all experiences have their place in the tapestry that is us, is a great exercise. It's far too easy to dismiss certain experiences as insignificant, when all experiences have been specifically selected for the person we are becoming. Carolyn Myss, a renowned spiritual intuitive, would even say they were selected by us before we were born into this life. I know I need to re-experience all my threads, the bright ones along with the dark ones, that have been woven into my tapestry and to point with pride to what is now a tapestry, still in the making, that at age seventy-one fills me with gratitude.

What threads of memories, whether tightly woven or unraveled, come to your mind as you read about my memories? Take a moment to jot some of them in your journal. It's my hope that you are beginning to see some of the beautiful threads that have been woven into a tapestry that's uniquely a reflection of you. And that the not-so-happy memories offer a clear contrast to those that are sweet, comforting, and worth their weight in gold as you sift and sort through the past that has made you who you are.

Sweet Times, Fudge, and Frozen Custard

One of the silly, lighthearted, but ever-so-sweet memories that always comes to mind when I think of my childhood is sitting on the living room rug with my mother and siblings and playing the Sorry board game that my younger brother loved. I can still hear his cackling laughter as he won yet another game, but the real joy of those occasional evenings together was eating my mother's fudge when the game was over. She created the most delicious, creamy, walnut-filled chocolate fudge you can imagine. We always knew fudge was on her agenda when she called us to the kitchen on a Saturday afternoon to help her shell the walnuts from our walnut tree that bordered the driveway. That was one job none of us tried to escape doing.

It was always a relief that her recipe made two pans of fudge, because we managed, every time, to completely finish off one pan on Saturday night. I can still see the pans she used; they were square with indented lines where the cuts needed to be made. I wish I had those pans in my possession. I can taste that fudge even now as I write these words. A delicious memory for sure.

I don't know why my dad didn't join us in those games, but he was on the sidelines, loving my brother's laughter, and he did share in the fudge. I do remember his presence within one frequent, good memory, however: the walk to the ballpark about four blocks from our home on many a summer evening. The Red Sox of Lafayette, Indiana, a minor league farm team that played there a few times a week, had the full support of my dad, so as a family, all who cared to join my mom and him could go to the games. His anger was sometimes present there too, usually when "our team" did something dumb. Whenever he got angry, I felt I needed to atone for it by changing his attitude or what I feared might be the attitude of others who saw him in that state of mind. My codependency was born at a very young age.

After the game, regardless of whether the Red Sox won or lost, we got the treat some of us had gone to the game for in the first place. We stopped at the Frozen Custard stand across the street from the ballpark. My dad loved hot-fudge sundaes, so it was sundaes all around, if you wanted one. I never turned one down. And I always chose hot fudge. As much as I didn't like my dad's anger, I did long to get his loving attention, so choosing to be like him, even when it meant eating smelly sardines spread on crackers smothered in mustard, was a common theme for me.

Decades later I learned that our little neighborhood Frozen Custard stand was famous for being a first of its kind. The *Wall Street Journal* had a front-page story about it and the family who had started it in the 1930s. That same family, the Kerkoffs, continues to own it and the hot-fudge sundaes remain as good as they were in my youth. I stop at the stand every summer when I'm back in Lafayette.

For much of my childhood, I was nauseated with uncertainty, even when my family was doing something as ordinary as having supper or taking a walk to the custard stand. Perhaps that's a common theme in families in which rage is the "ism." As an adult, particularly a recovering adult, I have come to perceive the similarities in all the isms. Families are held hostage by the one who is acting out, and it matters little whether alcohol, drugs, or rage precipitates the acting out. Waiting for the other shoe to drop is much more than a throwaway comment in families such as the one in which I grew up.

Sweetness in Logansport

I was able to escape the constant unease that existed in my family during wonderful two-week summer vacations at my grandparents' house. My grandmother and grandfather lived in Logansport, Indiana, about thirty-eight miles from Lafayette, well over an hour's trip in the days of two-lane highways. The trips to their house during the summer and on holidays are etched in my memory. I always sat nervously crammed in the back seat with my three siblings, trying to escape the smoke fumes from both parents' cigarettes, while my dad passed the slower cars in our lane. There were always slower cars, and as we were passing them, I was always afraid those cars speeding toward us were coming far too fast for my dad to safely get back into our own lane.

As a general practice, my dad swore a lot, but on those drives he yelled many choice words at the cars on the road, those slow ones in front of us and those speeding toward us. His swearing always embarrassed me, even if others didn't hear him. (And I was sure they could, since everyone had their windows down.) I somehow knew he didn't utter those words at work, but he did say them with relish in front of my friends, and I was often ashamed of him. The mother of one of my friends told me she had known my dad when they were both much younger, before he and my mother were married, and she had always found him handsome but was put off by his swearing. I wanted to disappear when she said that in front of a group of my friends at her home.

Arriving at my grandparents' house made the tense sixty-plus minutes in the car well worth it. Grandma was a loving woman, the stereotypical grandmother who always greeted us wearing a comfortable housedress. A little on the chunky side, she was always ready for our arrival with fresh cookies, cakes, and pies. I think she timed her baking to our arrival because the cookies were often still warm. Her chocolate-chip peanut-butter cookie could have won a Pillsbury Bake-Off prize. My favorite was her cherry pie, which she made with cherries she picked from her own tree. She even used leftover pie dough to make what she called *dolly vardens,* a special cinnamon-butter treat you'll not likely find in any cookbook, but we loved them.

But something even more special than these treats waited for us in the basement. My grandfather was the only candy distributor in Logansport, which meant any grocery, movie house, or gasoline station that sold candy— and in those days much of it was sold in nickel vending machines—came from Kirkpatrick's Candy Sales. He had only one rule: if we opened a fresh box of a favorite candy bar, and we each had a favorite, we were instructed to place the box on a table separate from the rest of the stacked boxes. We could take as much candy as we wanted, but we had to follow this one rule. He sold some of the candy in full boxes to the grocery stores, and he didn't want to sell a box only to discover it had twenty-three rather than the twenty-four bars it was supposed to have. We were diligent about this. My grandparents were so kind to us that we didn't want to disappoint them—ever.

As kids, we thought we had it made. And if the home-baked treats and all the candy bars we could eat weren't enough, there was a Frozen Custard stand right across the street. Every evening before bedtime, we all walked over and got a sundae, a cone, or a dish of our favorite flavor. Mine was chocolate. That was my grandmother's favorite too. No one I knew had it so good. What a relief no one was fussing over fat grams in the 1940s. It would have ruined it all.

I never heard any arguing at my grandparents' house, which meant I felt free of the tension that so troubled me at home. I never saw my grandfather drink, nor did my grandmother ever have more than one small highball at family gatherings. They weren't church-going people, except on special occasions, much like my parents, but they lived by the Golden Rule. It was relaxing to be in their presence, sitting on the front-porch swing in the evenings or going to the city park where we rode the merry-go-round again and again, reaching for the gold ring from the steel arm that was stretched out to us as we circled by it. Not until much later in life did it occur to me and my siblings that the reason one of us won the gold ring nearly every ride was that if one of us won my grandfather would pay for all of us to ride again. The man in charge of the merry-go-round was no fool.

When summer vacation at my grandparents' house came to an end, I knew the start of school was just a few weeks away and that I wouldn't get to my grandparents' home again until the holidays. That always made me sad, but starting school made me even sadder. Unlike many of my friends who couldn't wait to go back to school, I lived in fear—until I knew who my teacher was. Possibly having another teacher like Miss White, the second-grade teacher who tormented me with her mean stares and the point of her pencil in my scalp, prevented me from feeling much joy about the first day of school. Even seeing friends I had seen very little of over the summer didn't extinguish my fear.

Although after "graduating" from the second grade I never had as difficult a time with any other teacher, I was always nervous that my teachers would gauge my performance as worse than my sisters'. I was smart enough, but I didn't always have the best deportment. I was a talker and I vividly remember Miss Henderson in fourth grade making me stand in the corner, informing the class that I talked more in one day than either of my sisters had in a whole year. The class laughed and I fought back the tears.

A Special Holiday Memory

Any time we were with my grandparents in Logansport assured me of good memories, and I have hundreds of them neatly tucked away in my mind. One Christmas in particular, a good memory that culminated at their house actually began at my family's house the night before we went to Logansport. Until the day I die, I will cherish this experience, because it was actually free of the usual tension in our home.

My oldest sister, Jo Ann, was in charge of keeping my siblings and me upstairs until she was certain Santa had come. As is typical of children on the night before Christmas, we were eager and waiting on the stairs to go down to the living room to see what Santa had brought us. But she hurried us back to our bedrooms, certain that he had not come yet. I'll never forget her words: "Shhh, hear the reindeers' hoofs on the roof? We must get back in bed or Santa will not leave our presents." We raced back up the stairs into bed and waited. And waited. I, for one, did hear those hoofs. I was sure of it. My brother heard them too. To this day I can vividly see those images in my mind. For years I wanted what I was sure I had heard to be true. When the coast was clear, Jo Ann motioned that we could descend the stairs. Hurry we did, and of course, Mom and Dad were sitting on the couch waiting for our oohs and aahs, yawning as though they had just awakened. A successful Christmas.

The Christmas magic was alive in our house and in my grandparents' house too. When we arrived there a few hours later, carrying one favorite gift from Santa to show grandma, my grandfather met us at the door and said we had just missed Santa there. He told us Santa had stopped by to leave an envelope for each of us, an envelope he had forgotten to leave at our house the night before. Sure enough, my name was on the envelope my granddad gave me. He said Santa told him we could open them immediately. A brand new one-dollar bill was inside.

It's such a simple memory. But it reinforces the joy that comes from a few small experiences when you live with a childlike sense of anticipation, even when much of what you anticipate isn't joyful. I lost most of my hopeful anticipation as I grew a few years older, but knowing it was there at one time makes it easier to tell others on my journey now that the good memories still live in the recesses of our minds and that it's worth the effort to search them out. We need to balance the weight of the bad memories with the lightness of the good ones.

ू

YOUR TIME TO WRITE: Perhaps now is a good time for you to share some details of your early memories. Recalling the good along with the bad is the intent here. Think of this exercise as a form of pleasing yourself. Fond memories put us at ease. Not only are they good to recall but they are good to share with our friends and offspring. People need balance, and nearly every day we are confronted by situations that trigger us to anger or regret or resentment or fear. Quite likely any of these negative responses comes from a past memory that hasn't lost its grip on us. Having a body of fond memories from one's youth to resurrect at those moments can turn a bad day into a good one almost instantly.

I think it's wise for you to consider sharing some of these fond memories now, at this very moment, with a sponsor, a friend, a spouse, or one of your children—or better yet, all four. Sharing memories helps to solidify them in our minds. We have so deeply grooved our brains with the heart-wrenching memories that we have to expect the new grooves we are shaping will take some effort. We must see the whole of ourselves. Focusing on those defects that took us to places we now wish we'd never gone can and should be balanced by "the rest of who we were."

Write for a while. Share for an even longer while with someone. I'll still be here when you get back . . .

Here are some topics you might write about from your youth:

- *Did your family play any favorite games? Re-create the scenario of when you played them.*

- *Did you and your parents have specific activities that you shared on a regular basis? Describe those activities and what they mean to you now.*

- *Did any memories come to mind that "match" the one I shared about the ketchup fiasco with my dad?*

- *What brought the most joy to you and your siblings?*

- *Did your grandparents, on either side, play a big role in your childhood? Share some of those stories.*

- *If your grandparents didn't play much of a role, did your parents talk much about them?*

- *When you think of childhood aromas, what comes most quickly to your mind: your mother's cooking or someone else's?*

- *Do you have a collection of photos from childhood? If so, get them now and let them trigger memories you want to share here now, later, or with someone.*

UNDER THE RADAR, EVEN ONSTAGE

I loved school, for the most part. The exceptions came from being afraid of a teacher or an upcoming event—situations that were very real for me. But first things first: a few good memories about school. I turn to these first because they help me reframe—more honestly, I think—the less than favorable ones.

The good memories include the fact that I was a really good student (that is, until my college undergraduate years). I was an avid reader, and I loved writing stories, true as well as fictitious ones. Yet I never thought of myself as creative. My parents never acknowledged my creativity either. I'm not certain they even knew about it. Except for the Big Band sounds of the 1940s, the "arts" weren't especially valued in my family. I kept to myself as much as

23

possible while in the house, trying to stay "under the radar" I think. Being a reader and writer made that easy.

I envied my friends who went home from school and sat with their moms sharing the activities of the day over cookies and milk. I was thrilled on the days I was invited to join them. I had learned early on that sharing very little at home with my mom or dad was the wisest choice. There was little moral support for what anyone did; criticism for not doing something better was more often the norm. Now I have come to understand that people who feel they don't measure up can't comfortably praise others. They project on to us those negative feelings they have about themselves.

So as to not attract too much attention, I generally just did what seemed fun and easy to do and tried to slide by unnoticed. Lest you think my parents didn't love us, rest assured, they did. They just weren't able to express it in the ways I watched it being expressed in the homes of some of my friends.

In the sixth grade, my good friend Bonnie and I wrote plays and built a fairly elaborate stage from cardboard, construction paper, and paint. We made puppets from scraps of cloth, cotton balls, and popsicle sticks. We put on plays for the younger children at school. Did Bonnie come up with the idea or did I? I don't recall. It just seemed to evolve from our friendship and the fact that we both loved to read and write.

The teachers seemed pleased with us, and the younger

kids loved the plays. Of course, they all got to escape from whatever class they were in to see the play, a treat for the teacher as well as the kids. I loved the performances, pleasing the children, and ad-libbing lines when necessary. I can still picture the dingy room in the basement of our school where we gathered for the performances. The kids sat on the floor, and Bonnie and I crouched behind the stage. Might these experiences have planted the seed that has come to fruition in my professional life? Or did I come into this life with the seed already planted and the "assignment" to follow my bliss and let it create a major section of my life? It really doesn't matter, I guess. I simply know that from childhood on I have loved standing before an audience and sharing whatever words of wisdom have been passed on to me. The plays were complete fantasy, generally about youngsters involved in activities very much like our own. Usually there were good kids and a couple of bullies. The good kids always got praised for their behavior, while the bullies got expelled, or worse. What we were doing then relates to what I do now only in form, not content.

My desire to perform occasionally took on ugly overtones, particularly if I was intent on getting back at someone. And my dad was someone I frequently wanted to get back at when I was younger. His obvious disregard of my mother's feelings and the humiliation he caused my brother because of his poor reading skills and inability in sports made me seethe inside. I hurt for them both, and every time I had a chance to undermine my dad, I did.

Stomachaches

One incident stands out clearly in my mind. It's a rather long memory, but I think its inclusion is important because of what it says about my earlier inability to interpret people's actions and then forgive and forget them, knowing they were doing their best. I've had to work on acquiring these skills diligently for the last thirty-seven years.

In the second grade, during 1946, I was terrified most days. I was terrified of a teacher I was sure didn't like me, terrified of the point of her pencil against my scalp, terrified of classmates who made fun of me for having "four eyes" because I wore glasses, terrified of being called on when I didn't know the answers, and terrified because my parents didn't seem to understand or even care how scared I truly was.

Sundays were terrible days for me. I lay on the couch, tossing and turning, complaining of a stomachache, dreading the return to school the next day, all to my dad's very vocal displeasure. I begged my parents to move me out of Miss White's class, but they said no.

Then I began to have frequent and very intense stomachaches. Not your ordinary little upset stomachs, but deep inner pain. I complained but got little sympathy. My dad thought it was a ploy, similar to the one I had used before as an excuse not to go to school, and my mother was swayed by him, I guess, or too scared to disagree. Many days after walking the three and a half blocks to school, I had to go home. I was too sick to stay in the classroom. Fortunately my dad had already gone to work, and my mother let me stay at home.

Each time this happened, however, when he got home for lunch he severely scolded me and told me not to do it again. Then the stomachaches started affecting me every night. For three or four nights in a row, I got up and went to my mother's bedside and whispered that I was really sick. She'd accompany me to the bathroom to sit with me while I was doubled over in pain. My dad just got angry. The fifth night I got up even more frequently and my dad's patience had worn thin. Although my mother had walked me to the living room couch where she said I could rest, my dad said no. Upstairs I was sent, and I cried every step of the way.

The pain seemed to always subside a bit after one of these episodes, a fact that confirmed my dad's assessment that it was "all in my head." But then came night six or seven. A repeat performance was in the making and my dad had had it. When my mother went into the bathroom with me, he stormed in, pulled me off the toilet, spanked me with a book he had handy, and sent me off to bed. I cried myself to sleep. With all the effort I could muster, I tried to stay in school the next day but couldn't. I managed to walk home, intense stomach pain and all. While I lay on the couch kicking and writhing in pain, my mother called the doctor. Dr. Cole came immediately, took one look at me, diagnosed a rupturing appendix, and drove me to the hospital in his car.

My father was on the golf course that afternoon, so my mother was unable to reach him. When he returned home, he found her note saying she and I were at the hospital and that I was undergoing surgery. Needless to say, he was stunned and ashamed for doubting my pain. He rushed to my side, sat in silence, and was there when I woke up. I watched the tears stream down his face. The only thought I remember having was, *I got you!* Our dance was not a pretty one.

Learning Partners and Life Lessons

One reason for recounting this memory is its ongoing influence on me and my assessment of others. Even sixty-five years later, I may too quickly classify people—especially men—as being potential enemies if they are unsympathetic in a situation that is extremely real to me. Although it has helped me immeasurably to have adopted the spiritual philosophy that everyone on our path is a "learning partner," one who has been selected for the lessons both of us have come here to learn, I am capable of occasionally forgetting this and taking offense where none need be taken. I remain a work in progress.

The past, and our interpretation of it, too often determines how we look at the present. That's normal but, if our perception of the past is overly distorted and negative, it can impede our willingness to live our best in this moment. This moment is the only moment that actually counts in our personal evolution. For years, owing to the model handed down by Freud, no doubt, therapists have walked patients through their past. For years, some patients live in the recesses of their minds rather than in the light of this day.

I'm not a trained therapist and there may be times that delving into the past is good (in fact I experienced one myself), but staying there for months, or sometimes years, doesn't help a person celebrate or even appreciate what living here and now means. I'll return to my brief experiences with therapists later in the memoir. For now let me reiterate: living in the past under the direction of anyone doesn't guarantee that the "client" will awaken to the present where the next crucial lessons await us.

NOT AT HOME IN MY HOME

My hospital experience marked me in an interesting way. I was "the darling" of the surgical unit, a mere seven years old. Three other girls were in the room, all older, and because my grandparents had brought me a whole box of Hershey bars, I was very popular. The constant, positive attention I received affirmed me in a way that was unfamiliar. I had grown accustomed to either little attention or the more frequent negative attention at home. I wasn't all that undeserving of the latter. My easily hurt feelings prompted frequent pouting and lots of whining and even angry outbursts, not unlike my dad's.

I didn't feel at home in my family. I doubted, on occasion, that they were even my real parents. Part of this is owing to my overactive imagination, but living in a home where very few loving overtures were made was quite a contrast from what I saw happening in the homes of my friends. I didn't understand dysfunction then. I didn't understand the deadliness of fear and depression. I didn't have the labels for what I felt and observed others feeling. Home just seemed hollow and lonely. The silence was generally broken by the raised voice of my dad, a voice that was most likely criticizing one of us, mother included, for doing something "dumb." I can still hear my dad's voice calling my brother a "big dumbbell" for some tiny mistake. Those criticisms left a terrible mark on my brother, who had a nervous breakdown at age twenty-one.

I think my pain and loneliness tricked my mind into trying to catch these impostors pretending to be my parents on one of our many trips to Logansport. I hadn't fleshed out what I'd do if I were right, but stopping them in their tracks was the important thing. I began questioning them about events I clearly recalled from my childhood, ones that they had to know about if they were truly my parents. I don't think I really wanted them to remember the situations. I think, secretly, I hoped they *weren't* my actual parents. That could explain why I felt so outside the system. But they didn't miss a single recollection of mine. They could even supply details I'd forgotten. Impostors they were not.

I wish I had remembered to ask them about this when we all got older, after my recovery was secure and I was "reinstated" in the family. Would they have laughed or been hurt or figured it was just another example of my "creative" imagination? It's not likely they would have remembered, but the experience left its mark on me. I was to repeat this kind of questioning many times in my drinking years, as I searched to find out the details of what I might have done the previous night. I never got the relief I sought, however. My friends seldom remembered our antics either.

YOUR TIME TO WRITE: It's your turn to write and share with a loved one your recollections, perhaps ones that haunt you still or ones that clearly launched you in a positive direction for the next phase of your life. All of our experiences rest someplace on the launching pad. Being grateful for all of them is one of the joys of writing a memoir.

As in the previous writing session, scouring through some old photos can trigger many long buried memories. You might begin your search of the past with a specific recollection of something that happened with one of your parents, something that mystified you or was out of character for how you had seen them previously.

- *Were you ever in a position of doubting their love, their honesty, or their commitment to your well-being? If so, share some reflections to illustrate that.*

- *Did you, like me, ever try to "set them up" so you'd be vindicated for your judgments of them? The ego is fragile, and until we reach a point of comfort in the presence of a loving*

Higher Power, we are prone to do many insane things in our search for peace of mind. We can forgive ourselves for our past deeds, but we first must know what they are.

We are in no hurry. Write for as long as you like. Answers and peace of mind are what the search is about.

FALL CARNIVAL AND LOVE OF READING

Surprisingly, my mom and dad were quite active in select school activities, even though those didn't include coming to my performances as a playwright. My dad was president of the parent-teachers association (PTA); it was probably a necessity for the local banker to have civic involvement. Every year, Oakland Elementary School held a fall carnival, and it was a big deal. The fishing pond was always a hit. The prizes were simple and cheap but sought after. And then there was the cakewalk and the candy sale. Those two booths got the most attention. That wonderful fudge my mom made sold out first nearly every year. Her angel food cake for the cakewalk was always a favorite too. I always hoped I'd win it. Many years later, after being sober a few years, I tried her from-scratch recipe for angel food cake but failed to use pastry flour. My cake rose about an inch and looked like a big, flat doughnut. It got a lot of laughs at a party when I served it.

I can remember wishing every Friday night was as much fun as the fall-carnival Friday night. My parents were engaged and seemed to have fun; they left their critical voices at home. I discovered that other moms made really good cakes and fudge too, and my dad's sweet tooth ensured that we went home with a box full of candy, mostly fudge. We kids managed to make sure we carried home a cake or two as well.

My imagination remained vivid throughout grade school, and I loved both mysteries and biographies. Many of the stories I wrote during school hours or conjured up as a form of entertainment during my long walks home from my best friend's house had me as the protagonist searching out clues. I was much like Nancy Drew attempting to track down the man my friends and I were absolutely certain hid in the girl's bathroom at Oakland. Down dead-end hallways we ran, but he was never found. We could only hear his footsteps.

I'm not sure if this particular mystery-hunting activity reflected my fears or was bona fide creativity. But the recollection is worth savoring regardless. It pleases me to recall that writing was a real love even before it became my passion and my life's work. Perhaps I will be inspired to try my hand at fiction again one day. My story is still unfolding.

Not Fitting In

My memories aren't surfacing in a strictly chronological way. I think memories generally revisit us randomly. I want you to be comfortable with however your memories resurrect themselves. The past is seldom neat and tidy like the dresser drawers of a fastidious person. We really can't control which memory surfaces or when it comes, but we can get them on paper. The order isn't as important as the fleshing out of our lives so we can see where we were, where we are, and then evaluate those points along the way that hijacked us or moved us forward. Every experience plays an important role—every one!

Between being a playwright in sixth grade and taking my first drink of alcohol at age thirteen in eighth grade, my level of desperation about not fitting in escalated. The warm effects of that first drink of whiskey and Coca-Cola soothed my dis-ease instantly. That was both the good and the bad news. Had there been no payoff, I'd not have gone on to seek alcohol so often. But alcohol continued to give me relief for many years—until the day it finally quit.

What Happened

ॐ

VEERING TOWARD THE EDGE

Throughout high school, I had my share of sad experiences, but they were mostly in regard to an inattentive boyfriend and certain friendships with girls when I felt shunned. I wasn't bullied, thank goodness. I'm not sure I could have tolerated that. I had frequent thoughts about suicide over the simple disappointments of life. If I had had to contend with bullying, suicide would have seemed even more appealing. The feeling of being on the outside looking in, similar to how I felt in my family, was the most common theme. Then there are the all too vivid memories of excessive drinking and the dark alleys it began to carry me down, starting in my teens.

The Power of the Spoken Word

Within these recollections of my teen years are a few good memories, and I don't want these to be completely overshadowed by the ones that tug at me so vehemently.

I was a rather accomplished "orator." It surprises me to this day that I was a good public speaker in high school. As a matter of fact, the speech teacher groomed me for state competition, but I disappointed her by deciding not to do it at the last minute. I can't remember why I changed my mind. Certainly, I didn't take seriously whatever talent I had shown her in class. If I had to take a guess as to why I dropped out, it probably had to do with an issue entirely unrelated to speech class. More likely it was because of the boyfriend who took no interest in extracurricular activities. Codependency had been rearing its ugly head since my early childhood. Mine had become well-honed by high school, and whenever my boyfriend sought my presence, I ran to him.

At the same time, Mrs. Johnson, the advisor for the teen group at my church had gotten wind of my public speaking skills. She asked me about my willingness to "sermonize" before our large congregation. The assignment was to write and then give the sermon in our sanctuary at a regular Sunday service. I eagerly agreed to do it. Even though my parents were not regulars at Central Presbyterian Church, I knew they would attend on that particular Sunday.

I remember with some pride sitting in the beautiful church library doing the research and lovingly writing the sermon. Mrs. Johnson looked over my shoulder but made few suggestions. She trusted each of us scheduled to speak to say what was in our hearts. That, coupled with what my young mind surmised God would want me to say, made up the substance of the sermon I wrote. It was a challenge I loved.

And then the big day came. It was a cloudy Sunday. I half expected the crowd to be small at the service, but I was wrong. After the assistant pastor handled all of the preliminaries, I got the nod from Mrs. Johnson to walk to the pulpit. With a quiet and very sincere reverence, I began to speak, gazing around at the congregants as I did. I had already noted where my parents were sitting. And my siblings and aunt and uncle had come too. Although I didn't keep my eyes on them all of the time, I looked their way quite often.

I'm sure I must have read the sermon, at least in part. I don't remember. What I do remember, in fine detail, is coming to the close and raising my hand up toward the stained glass window to my left and saying, "God is waiting for us to notice his presence, at this *very* moment," and at that moment, at that *exact* moment, the sun shone through the window. The clouds had separated, allowing the sun to emerge, and flashes of colored light streaked across the sanctuary. The drama was palpable. I think from that moment on I was hooked by the power of the word, and by the power of God too, although that was not a communication thread that I was able to sustain completely. It was frayed, in fact, until far into my future. But I never fully forgot the immense power of His presence at that moment in time.

I didn't continue speaking in public, but I tucked away in my heart the joy of the experience, and I have recalled it on many occasions. One sidebar to the experience was my father's tears as he hugged me at the end of the service. Our relationship had few tender moments, and to this day I cherish that I was able to see the sensitive, loving side of him. And I'm certain it's not a coincidence that the seed for what I now do so lovingly and willingly was firmly planted when I was sixteen.

Beginning to Run Wilder

My public speaking was highlighted in a radio broadcasting class that my high school offered. Mr. Fraser, the teacher, was a fun man, younger than many of our teachers and perhaps too familiar with us. I'm not sure I ever got good at reading the news, because I didn't take the class very seriously, but I did take seriously Mr. Fraser's friendship. One way he demonstrated his friendship was to allow my friend and me to reach in his jacket pocket and remove cigarettes. Because he didn't personally hand them to us, he avoided getting into trouble, but, regardless, he played a part in the transgression.

Along with having the cigarettes to smoke, my friend and I had the keys to the athletic office because we were "runners" for the messages the director sent out. Quite pridefully, we'd open the windows on warm spring days and blow the cigarette smoke outside to the delight of our friends who were watching below. We never got caught, not even the time we sneaked some beer into the office and drank it in full view of our friends. Am I proud of this behavior more than five decades later? No, but it does indicate the person I was molding—one who was heading for a life on the edge.

ॐ

YOUR TIME TO WRITE: Now is a good time to withdraw for a spell, take a deep breath, and search your memory once again for experiences that either mirror mine, perhaps not in content but in form, or are triggered by what I have shared so far. This is your story. I'm only here to initiate your recollections and help you find the many threads that have been woven into your tapestry.

• *What do you remember specifically about certain teachers in junior high or high school?*

• *Did any of them choose to be extremely friendly with you and your friends?*

• *Were you a smoker or a drinker on the school premises? Did you suffer any consequences for any of your "edgy" behavior?*

• *Were you a ringleader or a follower? What do you remember most about that role?*

• *Did your parents ever find out then about the inappropriate behavior you are sharing in this memoir? If so, what was their reaction? Did it change you?*

Take all the time you need to reflect and write and share with others too. I won't go away. I'll be here when you get back. Moving forward together is what this part of the journey is all about.

Taking Tickets

Along with drinking and smoking in the high school athletic office, I was the ringleader for a scam at school baseball games. My plan was simple. I had thought of it at age twelve, while selling tickets at the kiddie Ferris wheel in our local park. I was the ticket seller and one of the boys in the sixth grade, a boy I had known since first grade, collected the tickets. One day, I not so innocently suggested that we resell some of the tickets he collected, which meant not tearing them in two. He agreed, and we often made an extra dollar or two on busy weekends.

This "program" translated nicely in high school, because a half dozen of my girlfriends and I handled the tickets at the hometown baseball games. A few of us sold the tickets and a few collected them at the gate. We succeeded quite nicely for a couple of months—until the director of sports administration, Mr. Lane, got suspicious about the receipts we turned in. He suspected that some of the money was disappearing because we were turning in too little money for the number of people present at the game. Unbeknownst to us, he had begun counting the number of people in the stands. When he compared that number to the ticket stubs we turned in, he knew something was amiss.

He came to us at the end of one of the next games and asked that we report to his office first thing Monday morning. We all knew he had gotten wise. And we all knew that the suggestion to steal had been mine. We hadn't pocketed much. Not more than two or three dollars per person per game, but it was outright theft, nonetheless.

I remember wanting to tell my folks over the weekend because I didn't want them to get a call from the school, but I was just too afraid to. And I remember being terrified that my friends would tell Mr. Lane that it had been my suggestion from the start. What an awful weekend. The shame and terror I felt made the financial gain seem very slim.

When Monday rolled around, I was the last to arrive at Mr. Lane's office, which made me very nervous. I was sure my friends had already "fingered" me. They had not. Mr. Lane looked sternly across his desk at all of us and said he should call our folks and have us expelled, but he wouldn't if we would tell him what had possessed us. At that point I took the blame and told him I had made the suggestion and my friends just followed along. He looked incredulously at me. And he threw in a bit of shame, telling me how disappointed my folks would be. How well I knew the truth of that. Then he said we were "relieved" of our ticket sales duties and no longer could we be the runners for messages from his office. He got up from his desk and walked out the door. We all continued to sit for a moment, then sheepishly got up and walked silently to our homerooms.

Did I learn a lesson? Kind of. But did I really absorb the gravity of the situation? I think not. I know that today a teenager would likely get expelled for such an action. That we all got to go on as though nothing had really happened was lucky perhaps, but it also allowed us to skirt the real meaning of honesty, reliability, and trustworthiness. Had our lives been altered, even slightly, as a result of our dishonesty, I for one might have made some better choices about any number of things later in life.

CONNECTING WITH MY MOM

Some sweet memories continue, thank goodness, although it seems easier to recall the painful ones that generally resulted from my poor choices. Their imprint runs deeper perhaps. But digging deeper yet has paid off for me, because it has shown me how my life was always more balanced than my memory of it is, which has given me a reason to think I may have misremembered some details of the many painful experiences. Just maybe I exaggerated those details and their accompanying pain as a way to hang on to resentment and to be unforgiving, defects that can fester and make any wound more infectious. I have discovered that hanging on to these defects infects all relationships, as a matter of course.

Even though I wasn't keen on going to college (I was far more interested in marrying my inattentive boyfriend and becoming a hairdresser), my mother convinced me college was a wise idea. Hairdressing, she said, could always be an alternate choice at a later date. Of course, she was right.

She had always hoped she could go to college when she was young, but finances didn't permit it. She wanted me to do what she hadn't been able to do, I think. I have often thought that likewise she secretly enjoyed my many battles with my dad, since she couldn't do battle with him. Was she living through me in a sense? I don't know. From my perspective, we didn't have much of a connection until later in our lives, but when that connection came, it was tender and ever so sweet, a part of my story I look forward to sharing with you. I see it as a way to honor her too, even though she has been gone since 1998. Gone, but remembered every day.

Pledging to Belong

In college, I wasn't a great student, really. It wasn't for lack of ability but because of inattention to classes and assignments. I was a party girl, and I found many others who wanted to party with me. But I also made some wonderful friends when I pledged a sorority, which was not something I had counted on doing. It pleased my parents, however, because it was the same sorority both of my sisters had been members of. There was definitely an upside to sorority life. It gave me a sense of belonging, unlike anything I had ever before experienced, and a taste of freedom.

Because I went to nearby Purdue University in West Lafayette, I was a "town girl," so I didn't move completely into the sorority house. Instead, I stayed in a separate dorm for those of us who still lived at home part-time. Living part-time in the sorority house allowed real freedom, more than I had ever been allowed. No one was looking over my shoulder seeking to know whom I was talking to on the phone, asking questions about my personal business, or checking up on my studies. The adventure in all of this was that no one, neither my parents nor the "house mother," knew for sure which nights I was supposed to be where. I certainly wasn't where I needed to be on many nights. Nor were my friends who signed out to my home and my unsuspecting parents when they wanted a little extra freedom.

One joy of sorority life was having a place to go after classes, being part of a group that seemed to really enjoy my presence, sitting at bridge tables and laughing until we cried, and then figuring out how to cover up for each other when house rules were broken, which was often, in my case.

I discovered that I had the courage to try many things that my friends thought too dangerous, although a few girls did follow my lead, reminiscent of those who had followed me into a brief life of crime reselling tickets in grade school and high school. Getting caught at a fraternity after hours meant social probation. So did bringing alcohol into the sorority. I didn't care. I think I rather enjoyed being the "naughty" girl. And social probation, which involved some public embarrassment, wasn't enough to dissuade me from my antics.

My naughtiness certainly escalated along with my drinking. On more than one occasion, my mother lied and said I was home when we both knew that wasn't the case. She was my protector. Was it to pay me back for trying so often to protect her from the verbal attacks of my dad? Perhaps. We never discussed it. Nor did she ever tell my dad what she had done for me.

WOMEN OF DISTINCTION

Two women I became close to at that time are still friends, and although they live on the West Coast, we manage to meet in some part of the world every year or two for a few days. Laughing again over the same memories we resurrect year after year never gets old. The connection is just too sweet to let die. Not losing touch with people who know a side of you from an earlier time in your life that few others do cultivates an intimacy not to be forsaken, much like the intimacy those of us on the recovery path develop with each other. It's having the witnesses every one of us needs throughout our life that are so meaningful.

In spite of my many indiscretions while in college and in the sorority, and there were many, that same sorority selected me to receive the honor of A Woman of Distinction in 2001. What makes this ironic is that they selected me for my work as an author and speaker on behalf of recovery from addictions, yet my own addiction had developed deep roots during my undergraduate years in that very sorority.

The woman who was the "house mother" for that sorority had put me on social probation more than once for the very behavior that gave rise to the work they now honored me for. Who could have guessed this would happen? God does have a sense of humor.

What a wonderful experience it was to share the before and after parts of my journey at the awards dinner in Washington D.C. Some in the audience were no doubt shocked by the details of my life, but they gave me a standing ovation regardless. How wise that God only shows us what lies just ahead. More will always be revealed when its time has come. The unexpected twists our lives take are what make them exciting. God is privy to every outcome ahead of its fruition. We must not forget this—ever. It means we will survive all those unexpected twists if we believe in the message as it comes to us.

Recalling these memories, both the fond ones and the more painful ones, including them in some detail, has been very beneficial to me. It has confirmed what I had always hoped to be true: some significantly good experiences are mixed in among the bad ones throughout my life. Too commonly, I focused on the negative ones, because I was looking for a reason to explain my alcoholism, my constant feelings of rejection, and my low self-esteem. I don't need to define myself in contrast to the many others who are journeying with me, but doing so becomes a hard habit to break. Most of us, after we find our way into recovery and do an inventory, begin to discover there is more good in our past than we had previously thought.

SKIPPING ACROSS KEYBOARDS

While in college, I never imagined I'd be a writer. I got an undergraduate degree from Purdue University and taught elementary school for eight years. I didn't really consider whether I wanted to do that as a lifelong career, but it was an easy choice, particularly after my college advisor indicated the main careers available to women in the late 1950s were nursing and teaching. Being a teacher was an obvious choice. By the time of my graduation, I was married, my husband Brad was headed to graduate school, and I needed a job that could support us. I put away my hope to work in the field of psychology and did what so many women did in the late 1950s and early 1960s. What would serve the marriage became my work, first choice or not. Evening martinis eased the disappointment.

I definitely didn't take the elementary education classes in which I was enrolled during my last year in college very seriously. As far as I was concerned, they were pretty rinky-dink and took very little effort, which was good because that allowed more time for my primary focus, drinking. Drinking and observing my husband's drinking too.

One of the required education classes was music. If you were seeking an Indiana teacher's license, and I was, you had to be able to play "America the Beautiful" and a song of your choice by the end of the term. I had never played the piano before. The closest that I had ever come to it was sitting in my best friend Mary Ellen's house when I was in the third grade while she got her piano lesson. Her teacher

47

was kind enough to give me a cardboard keyboard that I proudly laid on the windowsill. I would hit "the notes" right along with her. I took to practicing "my piano" religiously, much to my parents' amusement.

A cardboard keyboard is easier to play than the real thing. The college piano teacher, who worked with us in addition to the classroom professor, gave up on me and said that if I wasn't going to practice, she wasn't going to waste her time on me. That suited me just fine. The day of reckoning when I had to play for Professor Randall and the other students in the classroom was weeks off, so I continued my reckless living, expecting a miracle of some kind to occur. I envisioned being called on, sitting down at the piano, and miraculously playing my songs perfectly. Day after day I went into the classroom with that thought in mind.

I knew the other students had learned to play piano. They talked about it often. I simply never admitted what had happened between me and the teacher. However, I did begin to get nervous the day Professor Randall rolled a piano into the classroom and started calling out names at random. I was glad he wasn't going alphabetically, since my last name at the time was Hilty.

The weeks passed, we neared the end of the term, and the professor had not yet called my name. I knew it was only a matter of time, however, and butterflies in my stomach had replaced the earlier vision in my head of being able to sit down and miraculously play both songs. Every day when I walked into the classroom, I said a small prayer that I'd be skipped again that day. And then the last week of classes arrived. I knew my grace period was over. Professor Randall walked into the classroom and said he had an important announcement. Those of us who hadn't yet been called on were being given a "free pass" because he had received a very prestigious position to head up the music department at Indiana University. He had run out of time, and he was dismissing us for the remainder of the term.

MY MUSIC LESSON

I was stunned. I would get a teaching license, and I didn't have to face the shame of not being able to play. I never told any of my classmates the secret I was harboring. I feared someone would blow the whistle on me, and I needed to be able to teach. I received my payback, however, early in the first week as a teacher in the classroom. My first job began in 1962 in the Oakland Elementary School where I had attended as a child. And the principal for my first year as a teacher was Mr. Switzer, the same principal who had been there when I was a youngster, the same principal who, like my folks, wasn't very sympathetic to my struggles with Miss White, the second-grade teacher. Fortunately Miss White was no longer there. Had she been, however, I might have discovered a very sympathetic side to her, one I couldn't have fathomed when she stood next to my desk with her ruler poised to crack across my fingers. When Mr. Switzer retired the following year after I began teaching, Mr. Priest, my former sixth-grade teacher, became principal.

Because I had not learned to play the piano or even any of the chords, I pulled out the old record player that was in the classroom closet and searched for the records that accompanied the music book, records I knew existed. Fortunately, I found them and instructed the boys and girls to open their music books to the first selection. One of the girls, Julie, volunteered to play the piano for us, if I wanted, so I agreed. She said she knew all of the songs already.

With the help of two boys, I moved the old upright into the room. Julie sat down and began to play, quite proficiently too. The children and I began to sing. About halfway through the first song, Julie stopped playing, turned to me, and said rather snidely, "Mrs. Hilty, you can't even carry a tune." I was embarrassed and the kids snickered, adding to my embarrassment. I mouthed the words from then on, much the way I had been instructed to do while in college when my sorority was in the finals of a competition for the best vocal group on campus.

During those three years at Oakland, I also had plenty of opportunities to explore the girls' bathrooms and nary a man was observed, nor any footsteps heard. Perhaps he'd moved on after the foolish, far too suspicious girls had quit looking for him.

MARRIAGE AND CHANGING GEOGRAPHY

For the most part, my life in the classroom, both in Indiana and then in Minnesota, where my first husband Brad and

I moved so he could attend graduate school, contributes many good memories to my bank of recall, but they are greatly overshadowed by the sad ones created by being in a marriage that was alcoholic and emotionally abusive. The dysfunction in our marriage moved with us to Minnesota. A change in geography doesn't solve problems, and after twelve years of marriage and many troubled pregnancies, our marriage ended. I was ashamed and devastated, not because I loved him so desperately, but because of the rejection and my fear of what others would say about me and my failure "to keep a man."

During our marriage I sought even more solace in the alcohol that had become my constant, committed companion, one that had been present with me off and on since age thirteen. Alcohol had never rejected me, but the men I had drunk it with always did.

Death and Intensive Care

While married to Brad, in the midst of many alcoholic episodes, I had become pregnant more than a few times. None of the pregnancies had been planned or even wanted, but they happened. The first one was a few years after we had moved to Minneapolis. Brad and I had separated briefly and reconciled after a month or two. I should have known better, but I hadn't told my parents that we had split up and now I didn't have to. Soon thereafter I thought I was pregnant. The signs all pointed to my being pregnant but the doctors said no. I went to them twice, in fact, feeling certain I was. But they were unconvinced.

We went on a vacation with Brad's folks, pretending that all was well in our world. My physical discomfort was extreme throughout the vacation. After getting home, I went to the doctor for the third time and once again they gave me a pregnancy test that was negative. The following weekend we went to a party and drank to excess, not an unusual occurrence. Miraculously we made it home. Somehow, though, we always did. Midway through the night, I awoke in extreme pain from cramping deep in my abdomen. I couldn't stand up so I crawled to the bathroom where I passed out. I doubt that I even called out to my husband. He wouldn't have heard me anyway. Fortunately for me, he eventually woke up because he needed to go to the bathroom. He found me on the floor.

I suppose finding me there triggered the release of adrenalin, which may have cleared his mind. He carried me to the car, a small, red MGB convertible, and drove to the hospital. I was rushed into the emergency room and the real drama began.

As I lay there on the gurney, conscious of nothing around me, I faintly heard a voice say, "She is dead. There is no blood pressure." I distinctly recall wondering if it was normal to be able to hear people talking even though you were dead. And then another thought passed through my mind and it was about a movie I had recently seen in which a woman was in a coffin and the people around her were about to close the lid. She knew she was still alive but couldn't move or speak. She shed a tear, an onlooker saw it, and the funeral was halted. I wondered if what I was experiencing was akin to that.

And then there was nothing.

I woke up the next day in intensive care, totally confused. Brad was at my side. The doctor who had performed surgery came in and filled in the details. I had died, for all practical purposes. He had come into his office, which was right next to the emergency room, to get a book and heard the code-blue call. He ran into the room and recognized by the size of my abdomen the signs of an internal hemorrhage. He called for blood, and I was rushed to surgery immediately. I was given nine pints of blood and my life was saved. Unfortunately, the fallopian tube and the fetus that was in it could not be saved.

I have thought about that experience on many occasions. The fact that the doctor came in when he did is why I can sit here today and share my life story with you. I would have died had my fate been left to the staff in the ER, but God had another plan for me.

That very close call didn't save our marriage, nor did it prevent me from other pregnancies. Before our marriage officially ended, I had three more miscarried pregnancies and then another ectopic pregnancy, just as I was getting sober. In the mid-1970s, ectopic pregnancies meant the loss of the fallopian tube, which meant, in my case, no more pregnancies. I have searched my mind many times to see if I've failed to grieve a situation that was worthy of grief. I truly have no answer for this. I think I was too sick with the disease of alcoholism and the codependency to discern what my real feelings might have been. I have come to believe, however, that God's greater plan for me was to eventually create books, rather than children, and I can gratefully claim having given birth to more than two dozen books so far. And I'm not done yet. Unlike having babies, one is never too old to write another book. Praise be to God.

ॐ

YOUR TIME TO WRITE: Let's take another break here. The following are some ideas you might want to write about:

- *Talk about your educational background. Did you study what really interested you or did you, like me, choose something safe, something that promised a paycheck you could count on?*

- *Did you, as an adult, ever experience a major relationship breakup? Was there one thing that triggered it? Or many things? Were you prepared for it? How did you cope?*

- *Do you see the value now of both the relationship and its end?*

- *Did the experience strengthen you in ways you didn't expect at the time? Elaborate.*

- *Write a bit about the career that most intrigued you. Were you able to work in this field for as long as desired?*

- *What specifically happened that set you on a new course?*

- *Did you feel the presence of your Higher Power through the difficult periods, or did you struggle, assuming you were alone?*

New Directions

I'm not on a pity pot about my earlier life. It was what it was. In fact, I have come to believe that every drink I took and every drug I swallowed were leading me to this very point in time, a place that gives me a nearly constant sense of well-being. However, I'd be lying if I didn't say it took years of experiences in the rooms, both in AA and Al-Anon, and hours and hours with a sponsor and recovering friends to be able to honestly understand the necessity for that marriage—and for its end—in order for me to discover and then fulfill the passion that has burned at my core since those days. But I'm getting a bit ahead of myself.

With the marriage behind me, I began to explore a new direction for myself, not out of passion or because I had set a specific goal, but because I felt the need to prove to others, particularly my ex-husband's friends, that I was "more than" who they thought I was. In the pit of my stomach, and in the throes of my insecurity, I feared that being an elementary school teacher had not made me an interesting enough life partner. And without a partner, I felt like a nobody. I was desperate, in fact, to find a new one.

Although teaching is an honorable profession that I, for the most part, loved and was good at, I didn't fit in with the more educated crowd—and I desperately wanted to. I wanted to feel comfortable having deep discussions with graduate students about existentialism, capitalism, the philosophy of Kant or Kierkegaard—the kinds of conversations Brad and his friends had all the time around me, making me feel outside the fishbowl, that far-too-familiar perspective that harkened back to my years as a teenager. I saw this next phase of my life as the time to break out of the mold I had lounged in for so long.

Before my divorce, I had never considered going to graduate school, but I was out of other ideas for what to do next in my life. Perhaps some specific experience that I have long since forgotten pushed me to consider it. What I do know is that school, particularly the writing that was required, became the glue that began to patch my life together again. I was thoroughly surprised at the ease with which I moved through the requirements of both my master's and my doctorate programs in American Studies at the University of Minnesota. In those six years of classes, which included dozens of papers and a 300-page dissertation, I mysteriously lived on cloud nine. I felt transformed and surprisingly hopeful. Before I was even sober, I loved the life I was privy to while writing and while soaking up all the fascinating information in class. I even loved my life for long spells at a time.

Traveling into Darkness

The times in my life I wasn't so fond of related to the men I managed to snag in my web, a web that I kept spinning every night when I hit the streets of downtown Minneapolis. These men were not guys my family would have approved of. Actually, my family hadn't been fond of Brad either, probably a key reason I chose to hang out with him. They could see that his reckless, uncontrolled drinking was a problem, a fact that I chose to defend with the plea that "He will change. He's just insecure around you."

How wrong I was—not about his insecurity, but about his willingness to change. Without help, alcoholism doesn't let us off the hook, and throughout our twelve-year marriage, neither he nor I were open to real help. Once we had sought the services of a counselor. With the help of the Minnesota Multiphasic Personality Inventory (MMPI) personality test, the counselor discerned my suicidal tendencies. I didn't deny them. In fact I had harbored thoughts of suicide since childhood. They seemed the easy way out if the pain of my "invisibility" got to be too much. The counselor said suicidal thoughts were not normal. I didn't believe her. I was intent on harboring my thoughts in secret. They gave me comfort, in fact.

With Brad gone, I tried to stay on track with my life. But with the exception of the joy I found in classes and writing, my life was pretty unmanageable emotionally and devoid of any sense of solid well-being. Alcohol certainly helped to drown out the fear and uncertainty, and I sought good feelings outside the classroom in the attention I received in the bars I frequented. It wasn't all that difficult to get the attention either. My tight jeans, long hair, and cowboy boots were easy "hooks." And I loved knowing that. This was not a pretty part of my life, but those years have convinced me that my Higher Power was always watching out for me, whether I was conscious of Him or not.

The thought of the many times I drove home, barely able to see the road in front of me, still scares me. It didn't then, however. The extended journey to the dark side, a journey both dangerous and unexpected, not only didn't destroy me, it didn't even scare me. And I know now that I had to make that journey because of its preparation for the rest of my life, a life that was to eventually include the rooms of the fellowship.

My near-misses of other cars, probably pedestrians too, were owing to the grace of God. I have no doubt. I also have no doubt that I was being saved for the work that was next on my agenda. Otherwise, the many men who followed me home and shared my bed would not have been so willing to leave without causing some harm.

A Miraculous Near-Miss

It's truly a miracle that I lived such a reckless life unharmed. When I saw the movie *Looking for Mr. Goodbar* in 1977, only a year after I got sober, I knew that my life had mirrored that of the main character, Theresa. But I was luckier. I didn't die. I did take some perverse pleasure in having lived life on the edge, the very edge. (I still do, I must admit.) I have a friend who says, "If you aren't living on the edge, you are taking up too much space." The edge seemed to fit me, and my ego loved the thrill of it and the attention it drew to me. In fact, I've no doubt that my Harley motorcycle-riding days in the late 1990s and early 2000s were a leftover from my "edginess," and I was many years sober by then too.

Like Diane Keaton's role of Theresa in the movie, my life as a drunk appeared pretty schizophrenic. By day I was a straight-A graduate student, teaching a full load of classes in the General College at the University of Minnesota, but at night I wandered the streets, seeking drugs, thrills, and a man to go home with after the bars closed. How I managed to juggle all the balls remains a mystery. I choose to think now that God was catching most of them while my head was being turned by the attention of men who certainly didn't have my best interests at heart. In fact, a second psychiatrist I saw in the midst of my bruised emotions at Brad leaving me predicted that I would die at the hands of a jealous wife because of my wild ways with men who were already "spoken for." I laughed. He apologized.

I survived the many danger-tinged trips over the course of three or four years to the wrong side of town with the wrong men to participate in illegal activities; and I did so with a mindless kind of ease and even a modicum of grace. I carried this mindlessness with me to Europe, right after Brad and I split up, during a trip I took with my siblings and their spouses. Our parents had gone there the year before, and they wanted all of us to experience what they had seen. It was glorious, the few parts I remember—the very few parts.

To this day, every time my family and I get together, something comes up about that trip that I have very little recall of. I was mostly in a blackout, but I do remember going to some bars alone, without them, and dancing with strangers. I also remember having a clandestine one-night stand with the tour guide on my birthday. Walking on the edge had me in its grip for so many years. I sit amazed, to this day, that I came though it all. But I never doubt who got me through.

After the second ectopic "father unknown" pregnancy, my life began to take a necessary turn.

ई

YOUR TIME TO WRITE: Time to take another break, don't you think?

I hope you are yearning to capture some of your memories before they get away. They won't likely mirror mine, but they will be the threads that have brought you to where you are now. Savor them. Honor them. Share them with someone, if you like. But for certain, begin writing them down.

What's the first memory you have of drinking? Did it include friends you could trust or strangers you realize now were not very savory, like had been true for me?

What kinds of activities did you find yourself involved in that you'd never consider participating in now?

You might have some fond memories of the drinking days too, and that's normal. Share some of them if you like.

Being able to discern just how present one's Higher Power was, whether we "knew him" or not, is very important. It serves as a touch point for our knowing that He continues to live at our right hand. If you haven't thought about the many times your Higher Power "stepped in" when you needed Him, now is a good time to do so. Write about a few of those times.

Surprised to Be a Scholar

The ease with which I wrote became the detour that took me in a whole new and extremely unexpected direction even before I got sober. And what makes this so very special, and I think one of God's many "interventions" in my life, is that a couple decades later it became a way for my grandson and I to connect in a most intimate way, a story I'll save until a bit later.

In the meantime, writing became my lifeline, providing me with immeasurable joy and offering me a sense of purpose. I was amazed that paper after paper was returned with an A. I was even more amazed that professors considered my thoughts worthy of their attention. I had never experienced this before. Never. Not in my family, where I was the one who acted out, or in my marriage, where Brad dismissed many of my thoughts as sophomoric and superficial.

So to have professors respond so positively was suspect at first. My fear was that they'd discover, sooner rather than later, that I didn't really think very deeply and that my acceptance into graduate school had been a mistake, just as Brad had suspected. Even though our marriage had ended and he had moved on with his now-pregnant second wife,

I suspected that it was painful for him that I didn't struggle with the very requirements of the doctorate program that eventually flushed him out.

I was not a scholar. He was the scholar. I knew he was in the ninety-ninth percentile, but I still don't know what I scored on the graduate record exam to get in. However, I had perseverance, unyielding discipline, and an ease with the written word, a quality that was necessary, considering all the writing that was expected of us. It was as if the ideas and the words I needed for the papers and exams were waiting to tumble from the recesses of my mind, bypassing any self-conscious consideration or doubt. Since getting into recovery, I see these experiences that I so commonly had, *and still have,* as obvious examples of God doing for me what I could never have done for myself. In retrospect, and with deep gratitude and humility, I know that God has shown up every time I even nudged the door open a crack. I also firmly believe this will continue to be the case.

Nearing the Edge

But there was a time when none of this seemed true. Even though I was having success in school, my personal life was in shambles. You'll recall my reference to *Looking for Mr. Goodbar.* And even though my nightlife didn't affect my grades, it did begin to affect my teaching. Many mornings I awoke, fearful to face another class, another group of students who were looking to me for guidance and wisdom, neither of which I had the clarity to offer. My mind was often too clouded from the activities of the night before to remember where we had left off when we last faced each other. The alcohol, coupled with the amphetamines, twisted my ability to think clearly. And that inability scared me.

I had seen firsthand what happens to people whose brains get fried from doing the very things I was doing, and I vowed to quit. One day. One day soon. I didn't want to end up on a street corner panhandling like so many of them. But it wasn't until the woman who was assisting me in a literature class asked me if I felt okay that I was certain others could detect my confusion too. On that particular day, I had stopped in the middle of a sentence and simply stared at their faces, having no idea what I had just said or what I needed to say next. I dismissed the students quickly, hoping they hadn't noticed. They had. When they walked by me, I saw inescapable proof of their confusion was present on their faces.

That was the last time I swallowed a white cross, the street name for amphetamines on the corners I frequented, probably to the dismay of my supplier, a friend I had met on the West Bank by the university. I kept swallowing LSD on occasional weekends though, and drinking unending supplies of alcohol every night and most mornings, but I wasn't game for street-corner uppers anymore. For some reason, I was still able to keep up with my crazy schedule of classes, exams, papers, and teaching while living the street life that called to me nearly every day. I know now that I had a protector. My life was being orchestrated. My experiences, all of them, were the preparation for what I do now with such relish. Might I have veered too close to the edge to have ever slipped over? I wonder that on occasion. But it's a question that finally leads nowhere, similar to asking the proverbial questions *Why me? Why am I an alcoholic?* The answer for me has become "Just lucky, I guess."

DEPENDENT ON APPROVAL

I've already hinted at some of the dozens of not-so-pretty parts of my personal life throughout this period. Far too often I ended up in an unfamiliar part of town with people I didn't really know, eagerly participating in activities that would have deeply troubled my parents, many of the activities not legal. Alcohol's power over the willing mind is unyielding, however. And I went wherever others seemed to want me to go. How I could be so rational and responsible in some areas of my life and so completely dependent on the advances of unsavory men in equally unsavory situations is owing to one thing: an extreme case of codependent insecurity that was heightened by addiction to drugs and alcohol. It frightens me to this day how close I came to slipping over the edge. Others I knew did.

When I got my master's degree in American Studies, my dependence on the approval of others ironically pushed me to go even further in my education. Throughout my graduate school years, I "coupled" with many poor choices. This was to be expected, as my "picker" was lousy. But then so was my self-esteem. John, the man I tried to hang on to as I was finishing my master's degree, was moving to California and taking my ready drug supply with him. I had hoped he'd ask me to accompany him, much the way I had hoped my high school boyfriend would want to marry me. But John didn't ask me, and as I sat in his apartment, devastated once again while watching him pack, I called Noreen, my former roommate. John had approached her for sex after I left for class one morning, but I forgave him. It was either that or lose him, a common theme for me.

I told her I'd received the approval from my examining committee to pursue my doctorate. I had told the committee that I'd consider it, but I didn't really plan to do so, a fact I didn't share with Noreen at the time. I was waiting, of course, for John to react to my conversation with her. I had made sure he was within earshot and could hear every word. He remained quiet, but in his silence I heard the all too familiar rejection.

I began classes the next week. John was gone, although not forgotten. My phone bill was ready evidence of my constant calls to him, many not even taken by him but by a woman who had already taken my place in his life. I began the search for his replacement in earnest even though I still planned to visit him as soon as I could nail him to a date. I didn't have to look long. Bars were full of men just like him, men who lived on the edge, with poor work histories but great connections to the drug world. Men who were looking for easy women just like me. My supply would be handled and my nightlife too.

The next four years of classes were similar to the

previous two. Miraculously, I continued to be a star student with a perfect grade-point average and I managed to teach a full load of classes too. That alcohol and doctor-prescribed amphetamines fueled my courage and energy levels is certain. For the first time in my life, I felt like I belonged in this intellectual community I had carved out for myself. I didn't know, until much later, that I was absolutely addicted to both drugs and alcohol, and that without them, I'd still have felt like a square peg in a round hole.

CROSSING BOUNDARIES

Throughout those four years, I crossed many boundaries with students and my own married teachers, boundaries that should not have been crossed and would not have been crossed except that my judgment was greatly impaired by my drinking and drug use. It's really a shameful period in my life, and I still have many amends I should no doubt make. However, I don't even know how to track down those I may have hurt or ensnared in my web. Wives whom I didn't know and students I no longer even remember were targets of my thoughtlessness. Frankly, their names have been completely erased from my mind. Suffice it to say that when I finally got sober, my behavior changed. Not always my fantasies, but my behavior.

Not being able to make all of the amends from one's past can be haunting, I know. I have lain awake at night thinking about some of the people and relationships that I endangered. When I recall the psychiatrist's words—that I was likely to die at the hands of an angry woman because of my entrapment of her husband—I feel ashamed. I didn't set out to live this kind of life, but I did it so easily. And with so little thought of the others who would be hurt if they knew. Stolen kisses when a wife was in the other room and clandestine meetings at motels or my apartment were frequent occurrences. Some wives did find out about the indiscretions and, at the time, I was indifferent. I lived without a moral compass then. I am deeply grateful that I can no longer even conceive of living that way.

The choices I made for so many years may well have been related to the sexual violation I experienced from a distant relative during my childhood, a part of my past that I have never forgotten but never shared. Or my choices could be the result of my misguided attempts to punish my dad for his rage and the harm I felt he had caused my mother and brother. My dad hurt all of us, and even though I came to understand his pain and the anguish behind his behavior, at the time of my acting out I understood nothing but my own needs, which may have been to attack him and men in general.

I realize that even the choice of Brad as my first husband was an affront to my dad, and to my mom for that matter. His alcoholic outbursts at family gatherings and in public restaurants, even before we got married, brought embarrassment to them in front of their friends. I surely wasn't proud of his actions, but I wasn't going to let my parents decide whom I could marry.

In fact, we eloped to make certain we'd be in charge. Some months later we had a formal church wedding, one that the groom came to very drunk, and no one was ever informed about the elopement—well, until now that is. We had gone across state lines to Danville, Illinois, to make sure it was secret. The judge invited his assistant and her secretary to be the witnesses. I had spent the night at a girlfriend's house, and we left from there so my parents wouldn't get suspicious. I knew in my gut that the marriage was a mistake, but I didn't know how to avoid it at that point. I had already given him my word.

My involvement in politics in the 1960s, particularly the civil rights movement, and my shaming of my family for their noninvolvement as well as their judgment of me, was no doubt another attempt to get under their skin. But I didn't sit around thinking, *What can I do next that will upset them?* My actions were honest. I believed in what I was doing.

I was hardened to how my actions affected them or anyone else. And I know this was because of my own hurt and often ignored and misunderstood feelings. My family wasn't all that interested in my feelings. The baggage from my past was the ever-present initiator of years of insensitive and mean-spirited behavior. My family didn't deserve all that I heaped on them. My own view of life had changed, I think for the better, because of moving to a more liberal part of the country and teaching in an all black school in St. Paul, Minnesota, but "my enlightenment" didn't excuse my attacks on them for not sharing my opinions. What a blessing that this program of recovery includes the strong suggestion that we make amends for our past behavior. I did as I was told, and my family welcomed me with open arms, never shaming me for causing them pain.

I am grateful to have chosen to believe while on this continuing journey that the people I have needed to know, the family that was right for the growth I needed, and those men and women yet to enter my life have all been *prechosen by mutual agreement* for the richness of the tapestries we are weaving. This idea gives me a modicum of relief and a sought-after explanation for all that I experienced and all I put my family through. The pain of it all hasn't been lifted entirely, and may never be, but I now know that the events that happened didn't lack purpose.

ॐ

YOUR TIME TO WRITE: So that you, too, can gather gratitude for all that you have been learning from the "visitors" on your path, take time to remember their contributions. Like those on my path, they came bidden. Take all the time you need to reflect and write about your journey. Remember, it's the process, not the destination.

Begin by making a list of the people you specifically remember from childhood who influenced your behavior, either positively or negatively. Were they relatives, friends of the family, or strangers who "just happened to make an appearance"? As I've said on more than one occasion, I've become convinced that no one is an accidental visitor.

Study how these "visitors" pushed you in a direction you might not have chosen, whether it was good or bad. Share how you have grown from their presence and how you continued to honor their influence during your journey. Don't be shy about going deep within the recesses of a memory. Our best growth is waiting for us there.

WAYNE AND MY NATIVE AMERICAN STUDIES

My focus of study in graduate school was Native American culture. In American Studies, which is a multidisciplinary program, students are free to choose the area of focus that most intrigues them. The only limitation at the University of Minnesota was that credits be spread equally over five areas of study: American history, American literature, the fine arts, social sciences, and foreign civilization. This was perfect for me because I needed the latitude and the individualized attention this kind of program allowed.

I didn't enter graduate school with a spiritual program guiding me, but one of the first classes I served as an assistant in was American Indian Culture. I was instantly fascinated. The class and the students, the majority of whom were Native American, provided me with a spiritual framework that had been lacking my whole life. And the following year, because of a promotion, I was teaching this course myself. The combination of my own transformation and my preparation to teach this course made Native American Culture the obvious choice for my area of concentrated study. This meant that all classes I took could relate, in some way, to the Indian in America. Not all of them had to, but many of them did, and my dissertation topic, "The Portrayal of the American Indian Woman in a Select Group of American Novels," was definitely defined by this area of study.

The good that this choice did for me was offset by the bad choices I was soon making. Like any alcoholic, I gravitated toward the bars, and now I found bars where many contemporary Indians spent long hours drinking away their sorrows. Drinking with them, I observed firsthand the devastation of their lives. And I knew, as did they, that the dominant culture, my culture, contributed greatly to their devastation. Quite possibly, the shame I felt over their treatment, a shame I didn't have to claim but did, influenced my behavior. Certainly my alcoholism blossomed and the two, shame coupled with enough alcohol, influenced behavior that was, at the very least, beyond the pale of propriety.

My best drinking buddy at this time, and an occasional speaker for a class in race relations that I was teaching, was Wayne, a Winnebago Indian. His family did an intervention on him and he went into treatment. I felt betrayed. And even though I didn't help him "escape," I was relieved when he came knocking at my door with a bottle in hand. No alcoholic wants to lose her best drinking buddy to a life of sobriety. I had celebrated my thirty-fourth birthday with a woman I taught with at the university. After a lovely dinner and more than a few martinis, I went home and opened my apartment only to find Wayne waiting for me, a bottle of rum and a quart of Coca-Cola in hand. I quickly changed into casual attire and off to Cedar Lake on the west side of Minneapolis we went. We spent the night there, as far as I know, drinking the bottle dry. Where he disappeared to I never did discover. Nor do I know how I managed to get home. But I did. Many alcoholics do. I had gotten home many times quite mysteriously. And many of those times I awoke to find "a stranger" in my bed with me.

Wayne was eventually instrumental in my getting sober. After his family's attempt at intervention, however, Wayne never again attempted long-term sobriety, and for that I feel bad. When I finally got sober some years later, I tried to interest him in the journey, just as he had tried to interest me in it many years earlier, but he was no longer game. Eventually he was lost to us.

First Step on the Road to Recovery

After falling asleep on the couch and waking up to a sky that could have been either dawn or dusk, I called my dinner companion Toyce and asked her whether it was morning or evening. She was alarmed, to say the least. I laughed off her concern and was relieved to hear that I could go back to bed for a few hours of much-needed sleep. The next morning she eyed me rather strangely and timidly suggested that maybe I should consider going to Al-Anon. She said she had been married to an alcoholic, and she thought perhaps that

I was spending too much time with men who drank too much. I assured her I was fine but that I'd consider her suggestion. And to myself, I muttered, *Someday, perhaps.*

Bless her heart. I came to understand that Toyce didn't have the courage to confront me about my own drinking, so she did the next best thing. I didn't follow her suggestion, at least not then. I didn't follow it for some time, in fact, but the seed had been planted. My journey through the dark alleys with no-name men continued, but every time I saw my colleague, which was nearly every day, I was reminded by Toyce's silence that I had not yet done what I had promised to do.

I think of those days often and incredulously. How much longer I could have gone on burning the candle at both ends without some outside intervention is anyone's guess I suppose, but I was next drawn to John, a former student, who had been court-ordered to treatment. As his "partner," I attended family-member sessions. His counselor requested I not drink while involved in "the program" and also suggested that I go to Al-Anon. His counselor was quite adamant about it. So for the second time, I was receiving the same instruction. Because, and only because I didn't want to jeopardize the relationship with John, I agreed to go. Within the week I had found a meeting in my neighborhood at a church I'd never before attended.

It met on Thursdays at 7 p.m. It was within walking distance, but I drove in case I wanted to rush out before it was over. The last few days without alcohol had been difficult, but I didn't want to make it harder for John, and I did want

73

to comply with his counselor's strong suggestion about the changes I'd need to make. Earlier Wayne had told me his counselor labeled me a "co-alcoholic," which must have been the term used for "codependent" in the 1970s. In the back of my mind I knew I'd drink again, but not in John's presence. Not this early in the game at least.

As I entered the room with the Al-Anon sign on the door, I was surprised by the laughter, the number of people present, and the ease with which they greeted each other and me, even though they didn't know me. I felt ill at ease and confused about the posters hanging on the wall. The Twelve Steps and the Twelve Traditions felt like an intrusion on my way of seeing the world. I immediately doubted that this place could meet my needs. I had become quite certain that if others only did as I wanted them to, drank only the amount I suggested, and left our life plans up to me, that my life and theirs too would run smoothly.

I was quite uncomfortable the first part of the meeting. Everything I heard confused me. It was quite clear that these men and women were not seeking the control that I was hoping to master. And God played a much bigger role in their lives than I planned for Him to play in mine. They were gracious, however, and asked me to come back. They even sent me home with a small blue book: *One Day At a Time in Al-Anon.* I was eager to capture the essence of control, so I read the book from cover to cover as soon as I got home. The following Thursday, when they asked me how I was, I eagerly shared that I had finished the book and was just fine. They laughed. I didn't get the joke.

Surprisingly, I kept going—not because I was grasping the principles Al-Anon taught, but because I wanted to do whatever I thought would keep my relationship with John intact. I continued nursing it along, moment by painful moment. My worries never ceased, however. He never complied with his part of the plan the treatment center had suggested for us. He wasn't ready to be sober. Or honest. Or faithful. His interest in our relationship paled in comparison to his interest in alcohol and other women, but I refused to see the truth. The thought of another rejection was just too painful.

COUPLES COUNSELING

One suggestion John's counselor made was that we get involved in couples counseling. Of course I was eager for any help to save this "sinking ship." He feigned interest, but it was quickly evident that his commitment to me and sobriety and counseling was not serious. We had signed up for six sessions. I went to the first one fully expecting him to meet me there. He didn't. I was prepared to offer a great excuse, of course. I was skilled at making up excuses for the wayward men in my life. Because I didn't want their behavior to reflect badly on me, I painted scenarios that I was sure were convincing. I had written fiction as a youngster, remember?

The second session came and went too and no John. He missed the third, the fourth, the fifth, and the sixth as well.

I tried to act as though it didn't matter that he didn't show up. No one was convinced, however. I couldn't reveal how I really felt. My pride wouldn't let me. Also it would have shown that my great excuses for his absences were nothing but shams. On the last of the six sessions, the counselor asked if I'd consider telling the group more about me. During each of the other five sessions, first one couple then another had a chance to "tell their story." "We" were the last couple and since *we* was *me, alone,* I happily complied with a short version of "our" story:

I took my first drink at age thirteen and felt instant relief from the overwhelming insecurity that had dogged me since early childhood. I sought to spend time with friends who also drank and went to college with two things in mind: partying and finding a husband. I found both. I eventually found that my insecurities were no longer lessened by the alcohol. They were actually heightened. Of course, discovering that my husband was unfaithful, again and again, added to the insecurities. Adding drugs to the alcohol didn't help me or save the marriage.

After our divorce and my entry into graduate school, my life began to resemble "the loose woman about town." I managed, or so I thought, to keep many balls in the air at once. I was successful as a student and a college teacher and my nightlife was full. Dangerous, but full. I was John's instructor at the university and our relationship resulted from a one-night stand following an end-of-term class party at a campus bar. Drinking, his in particular, had been a problem from day one, but I was sure I could help him control it by controlling my own. He moved in with me shortly thereafter.

The other couples sat in stunned silence, waiting for the counselor to respond. I'm not certain what I expected her to say, but she began by saying it was hard for her to assess us as a couple since we had not appeared as a couple in the group. I was ashamed. And so angry at John at that moment. How could he have left me high and dry once again? What she said next surprised me greatly. She said she suspected that my problem was not just trying to control John's alcohol use, but that I had my own issues with it too. In fact, she said, "I think you may also be alcoholic." Her next question was directed at the group, not me. She asked if anyone would offer to take me to an AA meeting. Many hands went up.

I left the gathering surprisingly relieved. I felt like I was embarking on an adventure, not unlike taking a trip to an unknown destination. I didn't mention the meeting to John for the time being. I had seen little of him, in fact. His disappearance wasn't unusual, but everything about him continued to claim way too much of my attention. I didn't want the relationship to end, but I didn't know how to save it either. I waited patiently and with some anticipation until the following Monday, the day of the meeting I had agreed to attend.

STRUGGLING WITH THE FIRST STEP

I showed up on the steps by the church a bit early. I didn't want the "volunteers" to go in without me. Had they not shown up, I'd not likely have gone in by myself. I did notice that those who were rushing in for the 8 p.m. meeting appeared in good spirits. They were dressed well, not in scruffy clothes like I had imagined, and they were generally in groups, or at least in couples. My curiosity grew by the moment. Finally the three people from the group, one woman and two men, who had volunteered to take me arrived. They smiled and happily led me in. I was awestruck at what I observed. At least 200 people were gathered in a large room, most of them sitting in chairs but a few were sitting on tables around the outer edges of the group. A kitchen area held most of the smokers.

The meeting began with everybody standing and reciting the Serenity Prayer, a prayer I had heard at Al-Anon. It was solemn, with that many voices, and I was moved. And then the long process of reciting names began: I am (Name), and I'm an alcoholic. The "Hello, (Name)" response to each one took me by surprise. When it got to me, I simply said, "I am Karen, and I'm not sure what I am." Everyone said, "Hi, Karen," and I felt surprisingly welcomed. Since I was a newcomer, I was directed to go to the First Step group and I did, happy that there was a special place for the beginners.

I didn't know what to expect, so when individuals began talking about the struggle they had had with their powerlessness over alcohol, I wasn't so sure I was in the right place. I hadn't considered myself powerless. But then I had never seriously tried to quit either. I loved alcohol and the effects. I felt about alcohol much the way I felt about cigarettes. I couldn't seem to get enough of either. And all of my friends matched me per drink and cigarette. When it became my turn to talk, I said I wasn't sure if this was even where I belonged, that it had been suggested by a counselor. I did say that it felt good being there. And it did. The too-frequent feeling of not fitting in didn't apply here. I was very much at ease.

One thing I noticed from the moment I walked in was the large number of men, mostly good-looking ones, it seemed. What I had assumed would be true about those who went to AA wasn't true for this group. My misguided conception of what AA might be like resembled the meetings in the movie *The Days of Wine and Roses*. The people there were real down-and-outers. This was definitely not the case in this group!

I had the feeling that AA was perhaps a bit like Parents Without Partners. I had never been a parent so had not gone to any of those meetings, but I had friends who did and they often counted on finding a new partner relatively quickly. I decided that wasn't such a bad idea at all. John certainly wasn't proving to be a very reliable partner.

By the time the meeting ended, all the small groups meandered back into the large room where it all began. I didn't see the three people who had brought me to the meeting so I started toward the door. Just as I was getting ready to leave, a very attractive man approached me and said he had noticed I was a newcomer. Almost breathlessly I said, "Yes." He said, "Now you be sure and come back next week." I read this as a *sign*. He was hinting that he wanted to be my next relationship partner. I was sure of it. And was I relieved. All was not for naught.

YOUR TIME TO WRITE: This is a good stopping place for now. I hope that many of the experiences I have shared have triggered recollections in you. If that's not the case, get really quiet and meditate on one or two of your past relationships or any other part of your journey that involved drinking or using drugs—before you decided to seek a sober, more peaceful way to live. Take all the time you need. We are not in a hurry. There is no deadline. This is your life, after all.

What helps me with memories is to make a list of all the guys and gals I remember from particular decades of my life. You can go back to childhood if you want. Sometimes that gets the "juices" flowing. Then ask yourself these questions: Are the memories good? Or do they need to be revisited because there is some work to be done with a particular person? If there is work to be done, be grateful for the awareness. We can't fully heal if we haven't been willing to heal all of the "tears" in past relationships.

Begin writing down the details that come to mind. The more you write, the more the details will flood your mind.

Don't avoid writing about any detail. That it surfaced means it wants recognition. And every forward motion requires that the past be fully valued and left more holy.

The beauty of the memory search is that we discover many wonderful qualities that we buried a long time ago. They may have lain dormant, but they were never erased. Recognizing all of them validates the person we are.

Are you liking yourself more? The deeper we dig, the better we will look. Trust me.

A "Date" with Co-Sponsors

When I returned to that group the following week, was I in for a surprise. My knight in shining armor didn't come running up to me ready to sweep me off my feet when I entered, even though I was quite certain he saw me. He was in what looked like a serious conversation with another woman in fact, but I sashayed over to his corner anyway. As I stood on the periphery, he looked up and nodded, but that was all. My heart sank. He obviously had not spent the week, as I had, imagining the beauty of our developing relationship, the details of the marriage that would ensue, and the path we'd be on for the remainder of our lives. I was embarrassed and unprepared for the rejection. I sidled away before it became even more obvious to him what I was waiting for.

I'm not sure that the two women who approached me

actually saw what I had been up to or were simply used to seeing newcomers scanning the men in the room looking, as I obviously was, for a replacement of the last lost love. But Eileen and Kris made themselves known to me, and I was quickly relieved that I was no longer standing alone. They asked me to join them for dinner the following night, and I was delighted, although still somewhat chagrined by the rebuff I had received. We met at a German restaurant. After asking me a bit about my story, my reason for coming to AA (and frankly I still didn't have a very cogent answer), they shared where they were on this path of recovery. Then they expressed the real reason for the dinner.

They wanted to serve as my co-sponsors, at least until I asked someone on my own, and they were going to tell me how best to stay sober. I was eager to listen and learn, but I wasn't prepared for, and didn't like, the first thing they said: *no relationships with men for the first year.* That seemed unfair and very controlling, to say the least. They hardly knew me, and they shouldn't really take charge of my life. Should they? But they proceeded to justify the rule. They said that most women, and men too, come into AA or other Twelve Step groups too dependent on others for their feelings of self-worth. Of course, their dependency on alcohol or drugs was a given. This was true for me too. But surprisingly, my obsession to drink, which had been a daily occurrence for years, had been lifted, easily lifted, it seemed. Part of the recovery process is learning to know who we are, they said, and to like who we are, independent of others.

It made sense but seemed an unlikely path for me. Not

drinking felt far easier than not being in a relationship. I had never seen myself as independent of others. On the contrary, I had always defined myself in relationship to others, particularly men. And if the men I had clung to seemed pleased with me, I felt secure and "lovable." Learning who I was as a single person seemed like a daunting task. And truth be told, I thought it was unnecessary. Had it not been for Eileen and Kris and their constant inclusion of me in their social life with all the friends they had already made in AA, I'd probably not have been able to stay on the sober and relationship-free path they had charted for me.

It wasn't that I hadn't already had an inkling of the value of what they said. In fact, in 1971 while I was teaching Personal Writing in the General College of the University of Minnesota, I had assigned a book that had opened my eyes wide to the importance of having a "life of my own." The book was *Why Am I Afraid to Tell You Who I Am?* by John Powell, a Jesuit priest. In that book he shared a story that showed me just how far away I was from having my own life. The story goes like this: John Powell and his friend Sidney Harris, a New York journalist, strolled down the street on many a morning, always stopping to buy a paper from a vendor, the same vendor every day, and he was repeatedly rude. Powell asked Harris why he was always kind and a generous tipper when the fellow was always rude. His reply was the key: Why should I let him decide what kind of day I'm going to have?

I realized that I had lived my entire life at the mercy of others' treatment. Whatever was said to me, and how it was said, defined me for the day. I knew I could make a different choice but wasn't yet capable.

Steps in a New Direction

Now my new friends were in essence saying, "Yes, you can make other choices and, if you stick with us, we will show you how." I did just that. We went roller-skating, cross-country skiing, and played tennis. For many months, Eileen and I met every morning at 6 a.m. at the tennis courts in Loring Park, which were close to my Minneapolis apartment. Together we went to AA parties nearly every weekend. Even though I wanted to stray from my "agreement," I didn't.

I'm not sure why I didn't stray, but I imagine it was because I didn't want to disappoint these two women. They had taken such an interest in my recovery. I certainly had my sights on a few men, but I didn't pursue them and they didn't pursue me. Perhaps they could see the wayward signs of the too-eager woman in my eyes. Maybe that's what the first man had seen at that very first meeting. Or maybe God was simply saving me from the rash of mistakes I had been making all of my life.

I loved AA meetings. I couldn't get enough of them. And I so wanted to do "the program" successfully. For me, that meant "looking like I had it all together." I had so much to learn. So much. I tried to do some things too fast. Taking my first Fourth Step inventory was one of them. I didn't ask anyone how to do one. I just heard the word *inventory* and thought that meant writing down everything that had ever happened, much like in a memoir. And so I did. I wrote seventy-eight longhand pages of stuff: *what he did; what she said; etc.* In every scenario, I was the poor recipient of someone's unfair actions.

When I sat down to do the Fifth Step, again a process I was unsure of, I pulled out my seventy-eight pages and began to read. For four and a half hours I read and the kind minister listened. Or at least I think he did. At the end of the session, he gently suggested that I had done an inventory but not of me. I was devastated. I had failed. My need to do it right, or at least look good to the minister, hadn't succeeded.

Fortunately, I kept going to the meetings in spite of the shame I felt. Planning my schedule around them became a happy necessity, but I did still have teaching responsibilities at the university. As much as I loved teaching, I longed to skip that part of my life at times so I could just sit in meetings and hang out with my newfound friends.

COURAGE FOR CLASSES?

At the same time, I was beginning the fascinating task of planning my dissertation. My years of focus on Native American culture made my choice of what to write about simple. I loved history, literature, and the study of culture. Putting it all together in a detailed look at how the Indian woman had been portrayed in the American novels written by prominent white authors captivated me. Dr. Sibley, my dissertation advisor, was as intrigued as I was.

Before I got sober, I hadn't planned to keep my focus exclusively on white authors but my mentor, Dr. Roger Buffalohead, who was the head of the Indian Studies Department at the University of Minnesota, advised me to avoid including the works of nonwhite authors. His advice made sense. I had run into some problems already while teaching American Indian Culture. Most of my class of seventy-plus students were Native Americans. They weren't very happy that first day when they sauntered into the classroom. My white skin, long hair, tight jeans, and cowboy boots, not to mention the distinct look of the woman who drank too much, didn't impress them. That Dr. Buffalohead had helped me select what I included in the class syllabus didn't ease their cynicism. Nor did they appreciate that I often drank with some of their Native American friends.

Naturally, he began to hear the students' grumblings. Unbeknownst to me, he decided to pay a visit to the class. When I arrived on the first Monday of the next week, he was already present. I was stunned and assumed I was about to be "dismissed." However, his presence was to reprimand the class members. He assured them, in no uncertain terms, that I knew more than any of them knew about Native American culture, and if they were sensible, they'd settle down and begin listening to what I had to say. I was so thankful he had come.

Not a lot changed in the classroom. I never had their full attention, but I was no longer intimidated. I showed up, said what had to be said, and went on my way. It wasn't my only class, and I experienced great responses in some of the other classes. And I always had the end of the day to look forward to.

What a difficult period of life, overall, it had been. Without the alcohol to fuel my courage throughout the early 1970s, I would not have been able to show up every day to teach, to participate in my own graduate classes, or to flow through the hundreds of papers I wrote. God's availability to me, even though unappreciated, was doing for me what I could not have done on my own. The eventual appearance of John as a student in one of my classes, John who in a roundabout way initiated my recovery, has proven to me that God does show up in the most unexpected ways. It wasn't proper protocol for me to get involved with him, even on the last night of class, but I have grown to be very thankful that it happened. Sitting here now, writing this memoir, couldn't have happened any other way. I love the truth of that.

Abandoned and Hungering

I didn't really want to leave my old life completely behind when I committed to the AA program, and parts of it had to be continued. I was still a university instructor and a graduate student, but I couldn't rely on my old standby to get me over any humps. I quite surprisingly didn't hunger for alcohol or drugs, but I certainly missed the many people who had been such a big part of my life. That's no doubt why I was always on the search for the next "partner." Even though I did follow the advice of Eileen and Kris, I didn't stop scanning the crowd at meetings. Nor did I stop prancing around in tight jeans and cowboy boots. I was keeping a mental list of who might be ensnared in the future. In fact, the man who was to become my husband a few years later said the thing he noticed first about me was the "prancing." It hadn't been in vain.

Throughout my life, I was either in a relationship or searching for a partner. I didn't feel complete without one, and when I had one, I lived in terror that he would leave. Many did. I assumed all would. In the first year of recovery, I went to see a counselor my friends had recommended. I walked into her office, an office filled with dangling crystals, pillows on the floor, and burning incense. My first thought was to offer an excuse as to why I needed to reschedule. She seemed far too flaky to qualify for my needs. But before I got the words out, she invited me to have a seat on one of the pillows, and I did.

She was a gentle soul, very pretty, probably in her mid-forties, wearing a long, flowing skirt and a peasant blouse. She asked me what troubled me the most, and before I knew it I was telling her all about my fears of rejection, how it had happened repeatedly throughout my life, and my certainty that the pattern would be repeated again and again.

I began to cry and she moved over close to me, held me in her arms, and sat silently with me for a few minutes. Then she said in a soft voice that she believed I had been abandoned in my mother's womb. She said that my ongoing fear of abandonment was most likely rooted there. I cried quietly for a few more minutes and then felt certain, in a profound way, that she was right. My mother had abandoned me. But why? I didn't feel angry, just confused.

Revisiting My Family of Origin

During the brief period that I was seeing the counselor, I was also taking a Family of Origin class. I could see that many in the class knew far more about their parents' lives than I did, and I was eager to learn more. When the instructor gave us an assignment to interview our parents and other significant family members, I could hardly wait. I called my folks the next evening, explained that I was taking this class, and said I planned to come home soon so I could talk to them about their lives. They were nervous. I could tell by the way they hesitated. They weren't unwilling to meet with me, but I knew they weren't eager for this visit.

Within a couple of weeks, I found the time to get away for a long weekend. When I got home, I felt awkward. Neither my mom nor my dad seemed very much at ease with me either. I had caused so much disruption in their lives during my using years that I think they were afraid I was going to force some more discomfort on them. We had a very quiet dinner, and I think they were glad when I decided to turn in early to read.

The next morning they were both at the kitchen table when I got up. The picture window looked out on a very large green lawn dotted with bird feeders galore. The many squirrels fought the many birds for the seed and usually won, much to my mother's dismay. We drank coffee in relative silence. I announced that I was going out for a run but asked which one of them was willing to sit and talk to me first. My mother volunteered, and I was relieved. I changed into my running clothes and took off down the driveway, giving them time to wonder aloud to each other about the content of the discussions we were to have. When I got back, my dad's car was gone. He had temporarily escaped his fate. I went in and showered and then asked my mom where she'd like to talk. She suggested the living room.

She sat on the couch, and I sat on the chair next to the couch. She looked small and uncomfortable. She no longer smoked in the house because of my dad's emphysema, but I could tell she really wanted a cigarette right then. I actually wanted one too, even though I hadn't smoked for more than a year. I wanted to say, "Don't be afraid, Mom," but I refrained. Instead I said, "Tell me about your life, Mother." I wasn't ready for what came next. She began to cry. In fact, she cried audibly. Through her sobs she said she felt she hadn't been a good mother or a good wife. And then she said she was afraid she had caused my alcoholism *because she hadn't wanted me.* She hadn't wanted any more children when she found out she was pregnant with me because her first two pregnancies had been so difficult. *Bingo!*

The counselor had been right. I had been abandoned in the womb. I assured her, as I held her gently in my arms, that she hadn't caused anything and that she had been a perfect mother, exactly the mother I needed, a realization I had already come to understand from the many "elders" in AA. Together we sat for the next few minutes, saying nothing, just holding each other, and her tears at last subsided. We both wiped our eyes and then I said, "That wasn't so bad, was it?" And we laughed.

For the next hour or more we talked about the memories she had from her childhood and young adult life. She talked about the early years with my dad and his temper, along with his drinking too much on occasion. She never suggested he was alcoholic, and I don't think he was, but I was aware of his disgust with people who did drink too much—my many uncles, for instance. And certainly my first husband. My dad was of the mind that you had two or three drinks and then stopped, *"By God!"* Those were his exact words. He broke that rule himself only a few times. I always suspected that his anger was connected to his insistence on controlling how much he or anyone else drank. He would like to have "let loose" but couldn't allow it, and that pissed him off.

Mother and I talked about many more of her memories and it was a wonderful, freeing experience for both of us, an experience that opened the door to the kind of relationship many women never get to have with their mothers. She told me how she had hoped to go to college but it wasn't possible because there was no money for it. I think that's why she was so proud of me when I got my doctorate degree. Her letters to me were always addressed to Dr. Karen Sue Elliott (my maiden name). I think we lived through each other's successes. She learned to drive at fifty-two, and I learned to ride a motorcycle at fifty-two. She was proud of me, she said, just as I had been of her, but she was scared every time I got on my motorcycle. After she died, I "carried" her on my shoulder as my guardian angel every time I got on the bike.

During that visit, I had a chance to tell her how sorry I was for all that I had put her through and she simply squeezed my hand. I knew all was forgiven. We headed to the kitchen for a lunch of ham salad sandwiches, one of my favorite "at home" meals. I hoped the experience with my dad would go well too. I surely had received valuable information from my mom. I understood my own struggles better than ever before. I understood her struggles too. How alike we were in our insecurities, and yet, how brave we were.

After lunch, I asked my dad where he'd like to talk and he suggested the picnic table in the back yard. He carried his coffee cup outside with him. He seemed nervous, but he was often edgy. I opened up the conversation much like I had opened it up with my mom. I asked him to tell me about his life. I was as stunned by his immediate response as I had been by my mom's tears. He said that he had been afraid every day of his life. That he had gone to work as a bank officer every day filled with fear that he would approve a loan on a car, a house, or a business that the borrower would default on.

When I suggested that he would not have been responsible for someone else's failing, he slammed his coffee cup down hard on the table and said, "No, by God, it would have been my fault." I responded that people can make mistakes. Again, he angrily said, "No, by God, there's no room for mistakes in life." The hand that was not holding tight to the coffee cup was clenched in a fist, and I could see exactly why he was so hard on all of us. He truly believed in the need for perfection, and none of us was ever able to attain it.

Then I turned my attention to his childhood and asked him to tell me more about that. I hoped I'd be able to discern what had caused his obsession with perfection. And the reason came out very quickly. When he was barely five or six years of age, he was placed in charge of many chores at home while his parents were both working at a telegraph office. They worked in shifts generally, but one day they were both gone and my dad was in charge of mowing the lawn. His younger brother got his fingers in the way of the mower's blades and lost three of them before my dad realized what was happening. He paid dearly for his "mistake." I think at the moment he vowed to never allow himself to make another one.

The standard he held himself to was stringent. What he held the rest of us to was no less so. I understood, at long last, that his anger was really a mask for the deep-seated fear that drove his life. I don't think he ever told anyone else in our family about his fear. I think my mother died not really knowing who my dad was. I remember telling my siblings once about the conversation that he and I had had, and they were incredulous. I don't think they believed me. No one in the family was as comfortable with an expression of vulnerability this intimate as I was. Recovery had made the difference. My life relied on honesty and vulnerability then as well as now. It's an unchanging principle most of us in recovery live by.

After my visit home, I returned to Minneapolis with a new understanding of who I was. And for a time I felt relatively comfortable with my new life. I didn't continue to go to Al-Anon at that time because AA was consuming all my spare evenings. And I did spend as much time socially with my new friends as I could spare. Juggling all the balls wasn't easy, however. Meetings, teaching, grading papers, writing papers, planning my dissertation, and just hanging out with others, without alcohol as the glue, left little time for getting off track. And yet I did get off track in due time with the spiritual part of the program. As a matter of fact, I got way off track in that area. And my life began to feel scary and lonely. The isolation that is anathema to alcoholics became my constant companion.

LETTING GO

The change began shortly after my first AA birthday. It was as though a veil dropped between me and everyone else. In meetings I felt relatively connected, but once I got home, the comfort was gone. It seemed the dark cloud that had followed me so much during my younger years had caught up with me again. I woke with it and went to bed with it. It wasn't the companion I was longing for. Nor was I longing for God, even though I should have been. I didn't know how to find Him anymore. I'm not sure I had ever really found Him, even in the good days of early sobriety, but when I was with others who were happy, I felt happy too. At home alone, I was depressed and scared. Surprisingly I didn't want to drink, but thoughts of suicide, much like the thoughts I had harbored since childhood, took center stage in my mind. *Why not?* I kept thinking. *Why not?*

Even though a psychiatrist, Dr. Willow, had told me years earlier that suicidal thoughts were not normal, I doubted her words. I had resorted to thoughts of suicide in the tough times for so many years that they seemed normal to me. What was dogging my steps at that juncture of life certainly made thinking about suicide seductive once again. I wasn't scared. I was just tired of feeling alone. Bereft of hope once again, I didn't reach out to friends or a sponsor. I didn't want others to know how insecure I felt. And before the age of voice messaging or e-mail, it was easy to lie about calling my sponsor. She didn't have an answering machine on her phone either. I could *say* I reached out when I hadn't. No one was the wiser. Neither was I, of course. I was the one who suffered.

I withdrew more and more, day after day. My phone rang unanswered. I didn't call to report that I wasn't going to show up to teach my classes. My own course work was winding down, so I didn't have many classes to attend and only occasional meetings with my dissertation advisor. I wasn't even aware whether I had missed any of those. My awareness of the outside world grew dimmer and dimmer.

I'm not sure what triggered the final decision that "today was the day," but one morning I got up and blindly began stacking all my towels on the kitchen table. Methodically I began rolling them in the shape of bread loaves. I planned to turn on the gas stove, once the windowsills had been stuffed with the towels, and sit quietly in the kitchen until the gas lulled me into a deep sleep. I'm not sure I had thought this out very carefully. It just seemed a seamless way to do it. No mess. No sound. No reason for others to even come to the door. I have no recollection of feeling afraid or wondering how my actions would affect others. I certainly had no thoughts of God. It was the sensible way out of the state of hopelessness that had overwhelmed me. Of this I was certain.

As I took a last look around my kitchen, I heard footsteps outside my door and then the first knock. It startled me, and I didn't respond. I wasn't expecting anyone, so I sat very quietly, hoping and assuming the person would leave. But that wasn't the case. The knock came again, this time a bit louder than the first time. Still I sat, making no response. And then for the third time, the person knocked again and called my name. To my surprise, it was a woman's voice. Again she called my name. Her persistence was not welcome, but because of it, I finally answered. I didn't want the elderly woman who lived next door to become alarmed.

As I walked to the door I asked, "Who is there?"

"Pat," was the response. Mystified, I stood on one side of the door while she stood on the other. She said we had a meeting and she had other appointments scheduled after ours. Her voice sounded a bit impatient. I said I remembered no meeting, but she was insistent, so I opened the door, just a crack at first. There before me was a lovely, tall, red-haired woman I had never before seen. She appeared puzzled by my hesitation to open the door more fully so she pulled out her schedule book and, indeed, my name appeared on the page she pointed to. Our meeting was scheduled for 2:30 p.m. to discuss my financial plans for the future, she said.

I backed away and in she walked with an attitude of entitlement. She quickly made her way to the kitchen where the towels sat on the table. She looked back at me but said only, "Are you okay?" I muttered that I was feeling very depressed. I said nothing about the suicide plan, of course. Nor did she ask the purpose of the many towels. Her next question did surprise me, however. She asked me to tell her more specifically how I was feeling. I did. I explained a bit about my alcoholism and the dark cloud that had blocked out the sun. I didn't offer explicit details, but I found her easy to talk to. Her voice and demeanor had quickly changed the moment I had said I was depressed.

She nodded as I spoke. She assured me that she understood depression. She had experienced it, and so had her husband, who was a recovering alcoholic. The words she spoke next were incredulous to me: "I envy where you are." "But why?"—that's all I could think to say. My eyes wandered back to the waiting towels as I listened to her response.

Her explanation was specific and convincing. She said I was experiencing *chemicalization*, a term I had never heard before. She said it heralded a coming spiritual transformation. She assured me it was a real phenomenon that I could read more about in *The Dynamic Laws of Healing,* a book written by Catherine Ponder. Charles Fillmore, co-founder of the Unity Church, coined the term. According to Ponder, chemicalization is triggered when we are on the precipice of letting go of an old set of spiritual beliefs because we have been made ready for a new, much deeper spiritual awareness. She said the fearful ego was fighting for its life, however, and its life was tied to the former set of beliefs. The result was constant, inner turmoil and, for many, terror. That surely described my condition. Terror had me in its grip. Terror of the unknown. Terror about what was happening to me.

I sat at the kitchen table with Pat, both amazed and mesmerized by her words. She said I simply needed to "let go," that God was waiting for me to take His hand. The softness of her voice and demeanor stirred a change in me. She seemed so different from the woman who had nearly pushed her way through my door thirty minutes earlier. A calmness settled over me. In silence we sat and then she smiled, reached over and touched my hand, told me I was going to be just fine, and got up to leave. I stood and reached out to her. She gave me a gentle hug, put her coat on, and as we walked to the door, she said again, "Let go. He is waiting." She never mentioned the financial plan, the *supposed* reason she had come in the first place. Her business was obviously done. At the door, she again smiled and said I would be fine. I knew she was right.

I put the towels back where they belonged, poured myself a cup of coffee, and sat down at the kitchen table with a knowledge that I could, once again, face the world.

ॐ

YOUR TIME TO WRITE: Let's take another break here. I'm not sure if you have had an experience that matches this one of mine with Pat, but you surely have had one or more of those "critical, coincidental interventions" that took you down a different path, one that began to make sense in due time. Let your mind fully recall that time and place and follow the thread to where it leads you in regard to this present moment. Write to your heart's content. Include as many details as you possibly can.

- *Did you resist the "intervention" initially?*

- *How quickly did you discern that it was God making an appearance?*

- *When did you first realize what the real message of the experience was?*

- *How many times since then have you allowed that memory to comfort you?*

- *Interviewing my parents about their lives was far more fruitful than I had anticipated. Have you considered talking to your parents if they are still alive? If you haven't, please consider it. It will reward you immeasurably. Do it now or later. Just do it. And if they have already passed, interview one of their siblings, if possible.*

Take all the time you need for this exploration. It's extremely important for a deeper understanding of your own journey.

I'll be here when you return . . .

Spiritual Questioning and Reading

I have thought about Pat so many times since that day. I have even questioned my sanity. I never saw her again. Had I imagined her? Was she an angel sent to me, one no one else could have seen? It sounds a little crazy to even be posing these questions, I know. But it was an experience that, at the very least, was real to me, and it certainly saved my life. Had she not appeared, whether as an apparition or in the flesh, I'd not be alive to share my story now.

It did affect me in other ways too. I had doubted so many times whether the journey I was on was right for me—really necessary, I mean. I could see the value in not drinking (it made getting up in the morning easier), and I comfortably introduced myself as an alcoholic at meetings, but was it out of compliance? Did I really think I was alcoholic? Was

I fully convinced my life was unmanageable? I was accomplishing a lot, as a teacher and graduate student. Could I be doing all of this and actually be an alcoholic?

When I thought about Pat's explanation of my emotional condition, a condition I researched in the book she had mentioned, it gave me a sense of relief. Even though I had done much in my life, I had done most of it under extreme pressure that I had applied. I never let up on my intense discipline, perhaps because of my need to prove something to others or myself—or my dad. And in spite of it all, I did fall deeply into a hole of despair in the midst of this so-called success. The hole was closing in on me for days before I made the decision to opt out of this life. And Pat's words made the difference—all the difference that mattered.

I have shared this story in a public setting on occasion, when telling "my story," in hopes that someone might be helped by it, and many women have thanked me because of their own suicidal thoughts. We don't know which words we might say or what stories we might share that will make a difference in the lives of others. Did Pat know she was saving my life that day? I doubt it. But she was. What I choose to believe is that the God of her understanding and the God of mine had made a pact. It reminds me of Carolyn Myss's book *Sacred Contracts.* In Myss's book she explains that souls on the "other side" make contracts to work out issues in this earthly realm of experience. Once they have made the contract, they forget it, but the lesson will be presented. Never doubt that. I can only assume that it was part of Pat's "assignment" on this earth plane and mine too, to come together for the very important conversation that occurred. Our paths didn't need to cross again—and didn't. Our work was done.

Even though my emergency situation had been handled for the time being, I didn't live free of anxiety. It nipped at my heels almost daily, but I kept remembering Pat's words. My solution was spiritual, and I needed to let go and trust that God really "did have my back." I believed her words; I just didn't always put them to use. My anxiety continued to hound me. It didn't change much for many years, but I did hang on to life and sobriety. (I'll get to the precipitating factor that did bring about a profound change a bit later). For now, let me say that I kept my meeting schedule packed, spent time with my sober friends, and read spiritual books as often as possible. I generally began my day with one and closed the evening the same way. Even though I did all of this, the fear crept in far too often. I didn't contemplate suicide, though. I put pen to paper instead.

Among the many spiritual books I devoured in the early years was Richard Bach's *Illusions.* Because of his words on the back cover, I felt my life had to go forward. Since I no longer have the book, let me paraphrase what those words were: if you are reading these words now, it means you are still alive and thus have not yet fulfilled your purpose. That simple statement eased my mind the day I read it and on many days thereafter. I don't doubt for a minute that we each have a very particular purpose. Perhaps Bach's was to reach me with his words so I could one day write the many words I have written. We don't need to know exactly what our purpose is on any given day, just that there is one. Always.

For me, *The Road Less Traveled* by M. Scott Peck fell into the same category of books that Bach's was in. Both books, in their simplicity, gave me hope that my life was unfolding quite intentionally and under the purview of a loving God. These books gave me a reason to hang on. Every day for the first number of years of my recovery, I woke up with a feeling that the big black hole could snap me up at any minute. I had not forgotten Pat's words, and I knew my feelings were crazy, but they lingered anyway.

CODEPENDENT AGAIN?

Getting into a relationship, which I was finally "allowed" to do after one year in AA, didn't help anything. On the contrary, my fears escalated. The old obsession with *What is he thinking now?* wasn't gone. A year without a relationship hadn't healed that part of my insecurity. Letting him define me by his actions, his attitudes, or his opinions, even his facial expressions, was still second nature to me. I was flummoxed. I thought I'd gone beyond this infantile stage of spiritual development.

But codependency dies a slow death. If at all. As John Powell had so eloquently expressed when he shared Sidney Harris's reaction to a very rude newspaper vendor in *Why Am I Afraid to Tell You Who I Am?*, "Why should I let him decide what kind of day I'm going to have?" But here I was doing that very thing again. And again and again. It felt on many days that I had not grown at all. Actually, I hadn't grown much. And not at all when it came to being in relationship with a man. I have come to believe that the real healing we are born to experience is finally always done in the relationship dances we do.

Joe and I did recognize that being in a relationship would present particular challenges to us. We were committed to giving it a try anyway. With both of us on a spiritual path, we felt some assurance that we could weather the storms that might surface. And when we actually moved in together after a few months, we drew up a three-month binding contract. Neither party could shut down the relationship for three months regardless of the intensity of the battles. We knew the tendency would be to run, and we'd never know if we could succeed at relationships with anyone if we allowed ourselves to throw in the towel too soon.

So plug along we did. Because I was still so afraid of being rejected, I watched him like a hawk for any sign of impending rejection, assuming he might not really stick to our three-month contract. After all, he had never lived with a woman for more than twenty-two hours before this big experiment with me. At least I had had the experience of being married. It wasn't a healthy experience, but it was more than Joe had lived through.

It was probably fortuitous that in our first year together I was writing my dissertation, because that gave me something to focus on besides the relationship. I still managed to keep one eye on him, but the other eye was glued to the research and the writing that I so loved doing. Every day after my morning run, breakfast, and prayer and meditation time, I headed up the spiral staircase to my study and four hours of seclusion. It had been my decision to spend four hours at my desk every morning, whether I wrote five pages or two paragraphs. I instinctively knew that any piece of writing was put on paper one word at a time. I was doing it longhand and that felt good too. Part of me was merging into the paper with every pen stroke.

As the clock approached noon, I went downstairs, had lunch, and pursued any of the many activities I was involved with at that time. Balance and discipline came naturally to me. I've never quite understood why. Perhaps it's because of growing up in a family that stressed achievements. My mother had never worked outside of the home until my brother and I were in high school, but then she went to night school, learned bookkeeping, took a typing class, and promptly got a job. As a perfectionist, my dad became successful most likely because of his perseverance since he was not college educated. I had a sizable commitment to perseverance too.

Even though I was content and succeeding in some areas of my life, and I could look back on any number of "obvious" interventions by God on my behalf (still being alive was only the most obvious), I didn't rest easily in the belief that God was readily available. I still envied how easy it was for my friends, and Joe too, to access a Higher Power. I could catch a "glimpse" of His presence in a meeting or have a fleeting moment of awareness on rare occasions, but it didn't stick. Mostly I felt alone and anxious.

VISITING WITH GOD

More and more during those times of despair, I'd sit and "visit with God," mostly in the form of journaling. I'd escape to my favorite stuffed recliner, a brown, rather tattered chair that Joe's dad had given me. It was quite a struggle getting it into my study. Joe and a friend finally had to hoist it up over the railing of a balcony. In my study, I'd write and feel a presence unlike anything I had ever known, for two or three hours at a time on some days. This was my refuge.

But the well-being I felt in those hours didn't last. As soon as I rejoined the friends and family who loved me, my sense of separation from them was evident, and it wasn't caused by anything anyone did or said. I knew that, but I couldn't find a way through the veil. It simply hung there, with me on one side and everyone else on the other. But did I see a counselor? No. Did I talk to my sponsor? No. I could handle this, I was certain. I'd find the right book, one with all the answers I needed. One of Joe's sisters suggested that I read Emmett Fox. I devoured his words but found no sustained relief.

How do we maneuver through the troubled waters? My experience has convinced me that it's the hand of God and nothing else. Why I didn't attempt suicide again still mystifies me. The pain of my life was almost unbearable at certain points. In my search for peace, I eventually went through a family program for codependency. I didn't know how to have a life that wasn't enmeshed with someone else's life, a scenario that I cultivated. While in that treatment program, a counselor suggested I read *Love and Addiction* by Stanton Peele.

Like my experience with Emmett Fox, I devoured Peele's words. I knew they described my behavior. My desperation pushed me to adopt one of his simple suggestions: every time I was feeling insecure or "dismissed," I would retreat to the bathroom to assure myself that I was lovable. His suggestion seems too lame to have had the effect it had on me, but it got me over a major hurdle. My bathroom affirmation began to embolden me to retreat less and less in time. And finally I didn't need to retreat at all. I share this idea with others to this day. I think we have some experiences so that we can help someone else who is stumbling on his or her path.

Moments of Insanity

Even though Joe and I had made a contract to stay in the relationship regardless of the upheavals in the first few months, we strained the bond that held us together. Neither of us knew how a healthy relationship behaved. One instance early in our experiment of living together brought us to the brink of disaster and near dissolution.

We had added a temporary addition to the back of our home. We agreed that half would be his and half mine so we could each pursue our interests. There was an imaginary line down the middle, one we each envisioned. One morning while drinking coffee in my space, I took a look at his half and became incensed. I was suddenly certain that "his half" had crept over into mine, and I wanted it corrected. Immediately.

Joe didn't take my complaint seriously. In fact, he laughed at it. I seethed and began imagining how to get even. And then my eyes were maniacally drawn to the long picnic table on his side of our room. He had meticulously created an intricate mosaic on that table for an art class he was taking at the Minneapolis Institute of Arts. I looked at it with unseeing eyes and with one swoop of my hand, swept the hundreds, perhaps thousands, of tiny pieces of colored tile to the floor. They flew in every direction. He was stunned and initially speechless. I was too. It was a moment of insanity. My power of reason was absent, stolen. I knew there would be a repercussion.

Joe raced up the spiral staircase to my study, my "home away from home," and began dumping my file cases. My course work, papers, and personal business were strewn everywhere. I didn't know whether to scream obscenities or cry, so I picked up a camera and began taking pictures, announcing that I was going to mail the photos to his mom. And then we stopped. Thank God we stopped! Our moment of insanity was over.

I think what also happened in that instant was that we

each knew if we didn't back down our relationship would not survive. Wounded, we each retreated, but the more important response was that within the hour we asked for forgiveness. I no longer remember who asked first, but the healing was soon underway.

I can't really say that our relationship was based on undying love in those very early years. I'm not sure either one of us understood love. But we did understand alienation, and having felt isolated for so many years, we didn't want to retreat to that place ever again. Reaching out to each other, however tentatively at first, was far superior to pulling back and licking our wounds alone. To this day I am so grateful that we made that choice.

MIRACULOUSLY COMPLETING MY DISSERTATION

Every day, for the next few months, I kept plugging along on my dissertation while Joe kept himself busy rebuilding a 1936 Ford. As with every other writing assignment throughout graduate school, I ascended the stairs eagerly, every day. Something happened to me while sitting at the desk. Many times I sat back and looked at what I had just written and wondered where it had come from. The words almost seemed unfamiliar. I had heard novelists say that their characters generally determined the direction of the story, but I had never heard graduate students claim as much.

After a year of writing, I had finished the document. I

met my timeline and was happy with the outcome, but not entirely certain it was what others on the committee expected. Professor Sibley was pleased but he was a softie, and he had been reading it throughout the process. Five other professors had to approve it, and I had a much more distant relationship with each of them. I made five copies, an expensive endeavor for sure, and handed them out. Because the wait for the professors' responses was so anxiety provoking, Joe and I flew to California and then took a road trip up the coast. I stayed in touch with Dr. Sibley, and he alerted me to the approvals as they came in.

I didn't relax much on the vacation. My mind was consumed, wondering whether my work had measured up to the committee members' expectations. Maybe I'd "be found out." They could approve it with conditions, a scenario I dreaded. I knew others to whom this had happened. In fact, it wasn't that uncommon. The perpetual fear many students have is that they will be denied their degree after years of hard work. Would that happen to me? My first husband didn't wait around to see whether that would happen to him. And he had warned me that I shouldn't count on escaping it either. But he was out of my life, so I didn't have to deal with his constant judgment.

Joe and I returned to Minnesota, and I was pleased to find out that four of the five committee members had approved my dissertation glowingly. The one holdout didn't surprise me. Dr. Brown wasn't a happy man. In class, he usually groused and was often dismissive when any of us responded to his questions. In an American literature class I took, he skipped the inclusion of Emily Dickinson, which was on the syllabus and a main reason I had taken the class, giving the excuse that she wasn't really that important. That attitude revealed a lot about this man, I think. Having him as the lone holdout did not bode well.

I called him, hoping to find out whether he was close to the approval stage. He agreed to meet with me. My anxiety began to escalate. The day of the appointment, I awoke feeling nauseated. All the way to campus, I tried to think only positive thoughts, but I wasn't very successful. And when I got to his office, he sat, barely looking up when I entered. He didn't even suggest I have a seat. He simply said, "This has to be completely rewritten."

His words actually took my breath away. The experience that every graduate student dreads most was happening to me. I sat down across from him, uninvited, and said, "Dr. Brown, my orals are scheduled already, and they are only three weeks away. I surely don't have time to rewrite it." His reply shouldn't have surprised me.

"That's not my problem," he said.

The words that came out of my mouth next were from *someone else.* I was as surprised by them as he was, no doubt. "Would you consider going through the dissertation, pointing out the areas that trouble you, so I have an understanding of what needs to change?" I asked. He unsmilingly agreed. And that's when the miracle occurred, a miracle that has been unsurpassed to this day.

We started on page one and moved laboriously through the document to page three hundred, with him posing questions and me responding. For three and a half hours we conversed, or so it would have appeared to someone walking by his office. However, I heard nothing he said nor anything I said. To me, it felt like an out-of-body experience. I have never doubted that we sat there for that span of time, nor have I doubted that he asked questions and got responses. However, I have doubted that the person who sits here now writing this memoir was the one who responded to his questions.

When we reached the last page, Dr. Brown finally looked up over his little granny glasses, and said, "Well, I am satisfied. This receives my stamp of approval. I'll see you at the orals." With those words, which I did hear, he stood up, reached across the desk, and shook my hand. I walked out of his office, numb to the core, and went in search of a pay phone.

"Joe, you'll never guess what just happened. God showed up in the nick of time." That's exactly how it felt. Dr. Brown's criticism had reduced me to a feeling of complete surrender. I had been told by others on the recovery path that God will always answer us when we surrender our problems to him, but I had never been so trusting before. I had silently called out, and He had miraculously supplied the responses I needed to the questions Dr. Brown had posed. My next-to-last hurdle had been met.

Visualizing Success

My final hurdle was the orals, for many the most dreaded experience of all. It's a three-hour defense of one's dissertation before all of the committee members. We had all heard horror stories, of course, about a person freezing, unable to adequately defend even simple points that were raised. Not often, but occasionally, a doctorate degree was denied if a person was not "on his game," or so we were told. I'm certain not one of us took this event lightly. I had given it a lot of thought. A couple of weeks before my orals, quite by chance, I read an article in *Psychology Today* that soothed my fearful mind. Because I no longer believe in coincidences, I'm sure this article attracted my attention quite purposefully.

The topic was the power of imagery, of visualization. The author reported on a study that had recently been done with a group of skiers preparing for the 1976 Winter Olympics. One group of skiers had been taught to meditate and visualize their successful runs, the same runs they would be making throughout their competition. The other skiers spent their usual practice time on the mountain, skiing down the actual slopes, hopefully in record time. For many days the two groups prepared in this way and then the races began.

Those who had visualized their races fared better on the slopes than those who had actually practiced the runs. The explanation was this: when we visualize ourselves succeeding, we prepare ourselves to be confident. The day of reckoning is then met with success, not with fear of failure. The article's author wrote that the group who had visualized their practices reported feeling more prepared for their races than ever in the past.

I decided at the end of the article to put this information to my own test, and I began the daily practice of meditation, visualizing myself sitting around a table with six other people, including myself, in the room that adjoined the American Studies office. I watched myself nod to each one of them as "they spoke," and I watched myself reply, with a smile. For thirty minutes or so every day I sat in quiet visualization, feeling rested and a bit more confident each day.

And then the day of the oral exam arrived. As I dressed, I "saw" once again the scene I had been present at already in my mind. I drove myself to campus so I'd have alone time, and I still clearly remember walking down the hall to the exam office. I greeted Betty, the department secretary, with a quiet smile, and she nodded that I could enter. She mouthed, "Good luck."

I was surprised to see that all six of the committee members had already arrived. Even Dr. Brown was on time. The committee chair closed the door and the grilling began.

The experience was a repeat of what I had "seen" so many times already. They spoke and I replied. For nearly two and a half hours, we carried on a dialogue that was fun, relaxing, and successful. Dr. Sibley brought the questions to a close and asked me to step out of the room so they could discuss my "fate." After a very brief break, he opened the door once again and the committee members filed out, shaking my hand as they passed by. I was now Dr. Karen Sue Elliott. Betty was the first to give me a hug. The tears streamed down my face.

Graduation was a few months off because I had taken the orals in February, but the "let down" came immediately.

ॐ

YOUR TIME TO WRITE: This is a good place to "let down," I think. I do want you to consider some of the spiritual experiences in your early journey. Perhaps they didn't seem "spiritual" at the time but you recognize them as such now.

- *What was going on in your life at the time?*

- *Was there ever a time the words you needed simply appeared in your mind, as was true for me?*

- *Can you point to a few times you felt something going on that you had no real explanation for?*

- *Describe the most spiritual experience you had as a child, and then as an adult.*

- *Was there a single experience that convinced you that there must be a God? How has this knowledge changed you?*

Share anything else you want to regarding the spiritual realm.

On a Path Toward Serenity

I really wasn't prepared for the let down that came after my oral exam. I had been on one fast track or another for a decade, so filling the empty hours weighed heavily on me. I continued to write daily, even though the dissertation was now in the hands of the university. Writing soothed me; it was like a running commentary with the God of my understanding. That, plus the daily regimen of exercise, meditation, and meetings kept my life full and rich. Enjoying my friends, connecting with sponsees, and learning to be in a significant relationship kept me on my toes.

At the time, my relationship with God was definitely still a work in progress. Some days I felt connected, secure in the steps I was taking, and peaceful. And some days I longed for any indication that He was close at hand. Joe's mom always said that if God didn't feel close by, it wasn't because He had moved. I knew what she meant, but it wasn't all that helpful. And then she gave me a tiny little book that I savored like a good piece of Belgian chocolate: *The Practice of the Presence of God* by Brother Lawrence. It was a sliver of a book, really, but it held all the wisdom I needed. It was written centuries ago, but its message was and continues to be relevant to anyone who wants an intimate understanding of just how close God is to our every moment. I trusted that God was standing with me at the sink while I washed dishes, just as Brother Lawrence had written. God was there while I was peeling potatoes or making the bed. He was my shadow and it felt good.

"Practicing" God's presence changed my entire experience and understanding about God. The way Brother Lawrence spoke of God made a companion of Him, rather than a being who was somewhere off in the clouds.

This tiny book reminded me of Matthew Fox's *The Magical Mystical Bear,* a book I read during my first year of sobriety. In it Fox tells us to talk to God as we would any friend. Tell Him our troubles, how we're feeling, what good things happened recently. In that way, we will always feel a sense of His presence.

Both books gave a depth to my appreciation of God that had been lacking, a depth I had never been introduced to in my youth. I wanted to rest in the knowledge that God would always be "here" and wouldn't ever leave. In time I became certain that His presence was the only reason I was still alive. He had been by my side when I was too high to even consider his existence.

As I sat in my rather tattered recliner, having my daily chat with God, an exercise that I had come to cherish as much as a phone call from a good friend or a few moments of laughter with Joe, who was soon to be my husband, I sensed that our conversations were a bit one-sided. He spoke words of assurance. I mostly listened and wrote. Even the days I wasn't on edge with anxiety, which were few and far between, I sat and listened while He spoke. Eventually I developed a trust in His presence, a trust that has never left me, that is, not completely. The *knowing* that I now live with makes every experience just another piece of the tapestry that is my life.

THE COURSE TOWARD HAZELDEN

Following my big push to complete my dissertation and degree, I sought work as a writer in a number of agencies but was unsuccessful, so I looked for other kinds of work and wrote in my spare time. Writing helped me sustain my emotional balance. Then a friend suggested 1 seek work as a writer at Hazelden, the chemical-dependency treatment center and publishing house just north of the Twin Cities. Ironically, in my first year of sobriety, even before 1 had finished my degree, a woman who worked in research at Hazelden had approached me about writing articles for women's magazines. How she found me 1 don't remember. 1 had wanted the work but was intimidated by her deadline requirements and backed away.

When 1 approached Hazelden staff people this time, 1 was ready to be "their writer," but their answer was no— they weren't looking to hire any writers. 1 was offered a job, however—a job 1 had no preparation for. 1 took it, not certain why, but my "inner voice" spoke. By then 1 had learned to listen.

The first day on the job 1 was met with surprised faces. No one had expected me. The man who hired me had taken a few days off and had failed to inform anyone that 1 was coming. This greeting didn't bode well for me. 1 was led to an empty office. The man who took me there pointed to a stack of papers on the desk and said, "Your work is waiting." To say 1 felt anxious was an understatement. 1 called home and told Joe what had happened. He said perhaps it wasn't the right job for me. And yet 1 was curious. *Why had 1 been led here?*

That question directed my thoughts and attention for some time. My earliest sponsor had assured me that "Wherever you are, God is present and He brought you there."

The first time she had said it, I had snickered to myself under my breath. But no longer. Now I repeated her words to others too. I knew they were true. Too many experiences could be explained no other way. Remember Pat's visit just in the nick of time and my experience with my dissertation and Mr. Brown? Both of those events gave a richness to my life that continues to inform my every move.

Getting through that first week on the job with no boss was odd, but I've never been disappointed in my decision to stay. And my twelve years at Hazelden gave me many skills. I had a doctorate degree, but I knew nothing about management, production, marketing, or publishing. In my various positions over twelve years, I had to become a master of all four areas—without a mentor. One of my biggest problems was lacking the courage to ask the questions for which I needed answers. I didn't want others to know what I didn't know. This wasn't the first time I'd behaved this way in a job. This malady followed me wherever I went in my career. I could have used Google back then—daily.

But I did the next best thing. I hired people who had the skills I lacked and I forged a great team. For most of a decade, success was ours! It was as though no matter what idea we came up with, it struck gold.

My life wasn't without turmoil, but that turmoil wasn't necessarily job related. I continued to live with anxiety. It visited me as soon as I awoke and stayed most of the day. It took up residence in my body. I lived an hour's drive from Hazelden, which gave me ample time to pray, listen to spiritual tapes, and visualize the meetings that I knew were scheduled for the day. This preparation helped, but the gnawing in my gut was never entirely alleviated. It felt like hunger pangs, but I knew better. Food was not the remedy.

My writing continued to be the balm that soothed me most evenings. Following dinner or one of the many recovery meetings I went to, up the spiral stairs I'd go. It always felt like I was rejoining an old friend who had been patiently waiting for me. And until I paid a call, neither He nor I was peaceful. Of course, I realize how silly this may sound. God wasn't really waiting for me, but it comforted me to think He might be. Much the way it comforts me to envision my mother still "hanging out" in our living room.

The *unseen* is as important to me as the seen. I do believe in angels, and I think they are here to guide us. One of my favorite passages in the epilogue of *A Course in Miracles,* a book that was "heard" (it is believed that Jesus was speaking to her) and scribed (but not authored) by Helen Schucman, Ph.D., a clinical psychologist in the 1960s and early 1970s, makes reference to "hovering angels." Since coming to believe in them, my life has quieted considerably. Becoming a student of the spiritual path that is suggested in *A Course in Miracles* has strengthened tenfold my belief that there is, and always was, a greater Power in my life and I am being guided every moment. The "course" doesn't resonate with everyone. But the blending of it with the Twelve Steps of AA and Al-Anon has provided me with a steadier grounding than any one part alone.

A COURSE OF INNER PEACE

These days my anxiety is gone, and I experience a calm interior most of the time. To attain this state, I've had to surrender my will, no doubt thousands of times, to God. I have come to believe that had my inner calm come too quickly and too easily, I'd not have appreciated it so much. Nor would I protect it as I now do.

This is much the same way I feel about the study of any unfamiliar spiritual path. If reading about the practice explains it easily and completely, my tendency will be to put the book aside. If I am drawn to it again and again, because there are so many levels of meaning to be gleaned, my life will be far more richly rewarded.

This is, in fact, what my experience with *A Course in Miracles* has been like. For nearly twenty-five years, I have followed its included daily reading assignment, daily focused practice, and weekly discussion group. And I have barely scratched the surface of all that is there to be enjoyed in that book. For that I am truly grateful. Knowing that the "good things" in life never have to come to an end makes the daily experience of them like nibbles of one's favorite bread. We will be nourished and nurtured with every bite.

I have always felt the same way about AA and Al-Anon. Why would I ever choose to wander off when my life feels so complete, so gentle, so purposeful when I make time in my week to get to a few meetings? Meetings are not solely about us getting what we need. They are also about helping others get what they need. If no one showed up, the newcomer wouldn't attend another meeting. I think it's an obligation we have, one that I personally cherish.

My days at Hazelden were fruitful. My management team was stellar in every way. Although my boss promoted me, he didn't praise me or encourage me. I tried to treat my team the way I wish I had been treated. Just like with my dad, I grew to understand that this particular boss suffered from perfectionism as the result of fear. I think fear is always the underlying cause of bullying. And both men taught me great lessons. If you want respect, you must give it. If you want happy employees, you must praise. And if you want satisfied customers, you must do both. It's not rocket science. It's human relations.

The Question of Medication

Even though success sat at our doorstep at work, the anxiety that had taken up residence in my belly continued to plague me. I sought a doctor's help, and she suggested medication. In fact, she suggested it many times. I resisted. Again and again. I was certain that adding more meetings and exercising harder were the solutions, but the anxiety persisted. I had periods of reprieve, of course. During Twelve Step meetings and while sitting in my recliner with God at my right hand, I felt quite calm, peacefully certain that I was where I needed to be. It was during the many other hours during the day that my certainty wavered.

My husband is loving, but he didn't understand my struggle. Depression and anxiety like I experienced had never plagued him. His laughter came easily. His joy, upon arising, was evident. My life felt hard on so many days. I played subliminal tapes on my long drive to work nearly every day. My search for peace of mind and freedom from anxiety was unending. Prayer and meditation helped, as did the many meetings I attended. It was just all the hours in between that were hard.

I found myself arranging important meetings at work around when I thought I'd feel the strongest, the most peaceful. I'm quite certain that none of my colleagues knew about my inner turmoil. Well, perhaps my assistant knew. She understood so much and lent a helping hand whenever she could. But the mask I wore continued to protect me most days. For nearly twenty recovering years I lived in this darkness, always thinking that I'd someday discover the key to the happiness I observed in the many others around me. It was similar to magical thinking, much like the thinking I had when I was in college, expecting to be able to play the piano when called on even though I didn't know a note.

Had it not been for the writing, I'm not sure I could have stayed sober during this stage of my life. Too many hours of boredom, or worse, can be deadly to the alcoholic. That I clamored up the spiral staircase to sit in my tattered recliner night after night, for at least an hour or two, was my own form of prayer and meditation. It felt as though I called out and God answered—without fail. Much the way He answered when I called out when confronted by

Dr. Brown who said I had to rewrite my entire dissertation. When we call, God does respond. I have learned to never doubt this.

And yet, the darkness that shadowed me, that had shadowed me since childhood, wasn't alleviated except in small doses. I had talked to my doctor about it multiple times. We had talked about the family history of depression, both my dad's and my mother's. They never called it *depression,* but it was present. In spades. My doctor had suggested I try an antidepressant, but I refused to consider it. I heard from too many people in AA that any such medication was off limits. The attitude was that if you took something for depression, you were no longer considered "clean." I felt I needed to work my program harder, go to even more meetings, and pray more rigorously.

REGRESSION OR RELIEF?

After three years of listening to my doctor's evaluation of my condition at my annual checkup and hearing her finally say that she had prescribed an antidepressant for many other women in AA, none of whom had bad side effects, I finally relented. She promised that if I didn't feel better within four to six weeks, she'd look elsewhere for the answer to my depression. With trepidation, I filled the prescription, looking over my shoulder as I did. I was so concerned about what others would say if they knew. I was concerned about my husband's reaction too. He was so happy, so he really didn't understand depression. Like so many people (myself included), he thought that snapping out of it was surely possible.

The first morning I took a capsule, I had the feeling I had regressed. I was a failure. I couldn't do what so many others did with such ease. And I got no relief from the pill either. After a week I called my doctor and she reminded me that I needed to be patient. She said it often took four to six weeks for the relief she felt certain I would experience. I continued. Day after day. Capsule after capsule. I felt as though I were living a lie every time I was at a meeting. And what made it worse was that at nearly every meeting someone criticized doctors who prescribed medications that were off limits.

I so wished I knew some of the women to whom my doctor had prescribed antidepressants. I needed to talk, to get confirmation that I wasn't alone.

I was about to give up on the medication when, on day two of week four, I awoke with a feeling of lightness that I had never before experienced. *Never.* The darkness was gone. It was as though the black hole that had been hell-bent on swallowing me for so many years had finally closed. For a few moments I doubted the reality of my condition. How could I have felt so anxious and insecure for so many years and have it be gone this completely? I waited for the other shoe to drop. I waited. And I waited. But for the next few days, and the many weeks thereafter, weeks that have turned into years, my life has been on a different plane.

I certainly don't suggest the appropriateness of anti-depressants for others. Only a doctor can make that call, but I do believe that I'd not be sober, perhaps not even alive, had I not finally given in to my doctor's recommendation that medication was the necessary solution for a chronic condition like mine. I am so grateful to her for her persistence. And since then, I have spent the intervening years trying to be of service to others through my writing, speaking, and workshops. I have come to believe that every one of us has a talent and a way to fulfill it, if we allow God to have a say in our lives.

YOUR TIME TO WRITE: Let's take a breather here. Medications are not necessary for everyone. But if you have discovered relief with one, review your experiences. Did you fear the judgments of others?

What has been the most profound experience you have had with the God of your understanding?

If you have had more than one profound experience, and most of us have both before and after getting sober, take the time to relive and recount them. They really are the most important of all of our experiences.

If someone looks to you for help in connecting with a Higher Power, what's the first bit of advice that comes to your mind?

Do you believe in destiny? If so, what do you see as yours

currently? Are you content with it? If you had hoped for something different, why not write a letter to God, here and now? He will listen, you know.

The ideal is for us to feel passion for our lives and how they are unfolding. Do you experience that passion? How would you describe it to others. If you lack real passion for the experiences you are having, what might the solution be for you?

Was there a time in the past that you felt more "alive" than you do now? How might you reclaim some of that aliveness?

What's been the most surprising thing about your "newly acquired" spiritual understanding?

SUCCESS BEGUN IN DESPERATION

My life was different in certain respects after beginning the routine of taking an antidepressant every day, but I continued my long-standing practice of writing as a daily refuge. Quite surprisingly, I had met with a certain amount of success as a writer prior to following my doctor's advice. Those periods of untreated depression and anxiety had been fruitful. The publication and success of my first book, *Each Day a New Beginning: Daily Meditations for Women,* which became a best seller, was only the first of many fruits. Just because something is begun in desperation doesn't detract from its value to others, I guess. Even though it wasn't penned for the eyes of others, it eventually reached those eyes. As some would say, the rest is history.

I have been convinced every day since that first book was published that a miracle was made possible by "the intervention" of Harry Swift, the CEO of Hazelden at that time. I believe that God had intended this outcome as necessary to my journey, a journey that I am grateful is still unfolding and has included more than two dozen other books.

I'd like to share the backstory of Swift's involvement because of its importance. Swift was my boss's boss, and he and I talked quite often. He had shown a real interest in my work and was quick with praise. I told him about my love of writing and that I used it as a path to serenity and a connection to a Higher Power that I often felt far away from. I told him that I had originally applied to Hazelden for a job as a writer.

The more I shared about my writing, the more interested he became, and I eventually showed him the collection of "meditations" I had been writing for more than a year. His interest in publishing them as a book for women thrilled and surprised me. There were a few hurdles to overcome, however. My own boss wasn't so sure a book for women was necessary. Nor were the many other men on staff. And besides, *Twenty-Four Hours a Day,* Hazelden's first and best-selling book, had been "the bible" for decades. I took a backseat in the discussions and watched as the drama unfolded.

Eventually, after thirty or more women had reviewed the meditations and given them a "thumbs up," the boss said okay. *Each Day a New Beginning* became a reality. Hazelden released the book in December 1982. The management group had been quite certain that it would have a short life, perhaps no real life at all. They ordered a first print run of 10,000 copies, which sold out before the books even reached the warehouse. I was as surprised as anyone. I had no idea that my conversations with God would speak to any other woman. The same has remained true for me with every single book I've ever had published. I know that staying out of God's way is the process. He will show up if I move aside. I have been moving aside now for many years and many books, and it makes my life pretty comfortable.

With frequency I think back to that first book with tenderness and awe. I had no idea God was working in my life beyond the daily connection we had while I was writing. I was desperate and had to write daily if I wanted to feel any sense of well-being. No matter where I was, writing became my first priority.

We had a small cabin in northern Minnesota and on the dock I sat for many an afternoon absorbed in my process. On one afternoon, Joe was putting screens on the windows and wanted my help. When I yelled up to him that I needed to write, all hell broke loose. How was he to know, or me either, that I was writing a book that would sell millions of copies over the years. His retort at the time was, "Every woman I ever knew thought she was writing a book. What makes yours different?"

We laugh about that now. However, I was committed to my process and all who visited us, at home or at the cabin, could see that. I didn't realize that I was writing a book that others would ever read. I just knew that writing called to me and that I had to answer. On weekends when we had friends at the cabin with us, I set my alarm and got up early, hid out in the small shed behind the cabin that was originally built, but never used, as an outhouse. Fortunately we had plumbing, but the little shed served me well in another way. Sitting in it, I had a couple of hours of quiet time to write before anyone else got up, and that time alone with God, my legal pad, and a pen prepared me to be "right-minded" for the day. For me, there is a thin line between writing and meditation. My mind was and continues to be made peaceful by writing.

The health of my relationships is, no doubt, the main reason I continue to write, regardless of where I am. The well-being of all my relationships relies on it. Meditation is different for everyone. Writing is the most accessible form of meditation for me. Blogging has also been particularly good because it's a short form of meditation. I sit, God directs, and in an hour or less my mind is settled and peace has come.

I never imagined I could have a quiet, settled mind. From childhood on, my mind was constantly searching for indications from others that everything was okay and, in particular, that I would not be rejected. Now, none of those things that haunted me for decades ever cross my mind. With God's help I finally turned that corner.

Opportunity to Surrender

It was an unusual relationship I had with Hazelden. I was an executive within the organization, part of the team that determined the direction the foundation needed to take each year, and an author for the publishing division. The two roles didn't conflict. One activity usually occurred at night, in the confines of my study in our home in Richfield, Minnesota, during the writing/meditation experience that had become so necessary to me. The other role was fulfilled by day, in Center City, Minnesota, or wherever I might be traveling for the foundation at the time. I felt extremely lucky. And directed. But it wasn't until I resigned from Hazelden to commit my life to being a full-time writer that I got "in touch" with how very necessary my work at Hazelden had been.

To clarify, because of Hazelden and my boss there for the first few years, I turned once again to Al-Anon as a lifeline to serenity. Just as I did during the first forty years of my life, while I worked at Hazelden I had been letting the actions of others, such as my boss, determine how I acted, felt, and saw myself on a minute-by-minute basis. In Al-Anon, I was reminded once again, just as in the first year I attended recovery meetings, that what others did didn't need to affect me at all. And that no matter what they did, *they* were out of my control. I needed to be "a double winner." I was simply not capable of claiming a peaceful life for myself with AA alone; I needed the fellowship of Al-Anon too. And I'm grateful for that fact. With the two programs for most of the last thirty years, I have grown exponentially. At least that's how I see it.

It was during my tenure there in the 1980s that Hazelden began to flourish as the publisher of books for the treatment and recovery market. I can't claim credit for that. It was simply the times we were living in. Treatment centers were opening up around the country, even throughout the world, nearly on a daily basis. There were literally thousands of them in the 1980s. Hazelden Foundation's treatment center in Center City had opened its doors in 1949 and was considered by many to be the granddaddy of them all. It surely became the gold standard and the training ground for thousands, maybe tens of thousands, of counselors over the years.

The first collection of Hazelden books that the chain bookstores wanted to sell were the daily meditation books. We were more than happy to accommodate them. It introduced our titles and our way of thinking to millions of people who might not have discovered Hazelden otherwise. What a feather in our caps that entire endeavor became.

When I decided to leave after a dozen years with this remarkable organization, I felt like my work as a writer had pushed its way too deep into the center of my life, and age and energy didn't allow me to do justice to both "jobs." After a few short years away, I was invited to join the foundation as a trustee and was on the board for nine years, a level of involvement I found very rewarding. I am still involved with Hazelden in various capacities, both while in

Minnesota and also in Naples, Florida, where I spend the winter months. With certainty, I will remain loyal to them until the day I die.

When I left Hazelden, I hadn't yet started taking the antidepressants. If anything, my depression and anxiety worsened right after I left, no doubt because I had more hours in the day to be haunted by the shadow that followed me everywhere. But many good things came when I did at last relent and follow the suggestion of my doctor. Freedom from the depression was only one of them. I felt more eager to write, and it was not because I had to write to connect with God to feel okay, but because I wanted to. By then my relationship with God was tight. And it has remained so ever since, even though on occasion I have to give myself a nudge to count my blessings as proof that He has always been here.

I very recently shared the short version of my story at an event and was reminded once again that God was very busy on my behalf for many years. He still is, of course. But the key message I shared was that God is waiting for our willingness to surrender as the sign that we really want His help. But surrendering is not so easy. It's far more natural for most of us, in or out of this program, to think that our problems are ours to resolve. Alone. As proof that we are worthy, perhaps. Having a problem feel as big as the terrifying experience I had when Dr. Brown told me I had to rewrite my dissertation is what pushed me to surrender the first time. I have never fought against the opportunity to surrender since then. It makes every experience manageable. But even more than that, it has made every experience far more understandable in the bigger picture called life.

Gathering Wisdom

After leaving my job at Hazelden in the summer of 1990, I felt a bit lost. Who was I? I didn't have a full schedule of meetings any more. People were not looking to me for leadership, new product ideas, or conflict resolution. I wondered if leaving a job I loved so much had been the right decision after all, but my position had already been filled by someone else. There was no going back. My doctor had warned me that the adjustment might be difficult. I wasn't really a workaholic, but I was filled with the sense of doing God's will every day while I was working for Hazelden. After leaving, it was back to my old will, which was not a good place to be.

It was then that my husband suggested I consider exploring what others did after retirement, and another book was conceived.

Joe and I had already chosen Naples, Florida, as a place we wanted to live, not just because of the weather, but because of the nearly 300 AA meetings held there every week. I was extremely pleased with the Al-Anon meetings too and have been "at home" there in both groups since 1990. We found a small home we liked that included as an amenity a challenging but not excessively long golf course, and we have been satisfied with our choice of "winter living" ever since. We pack up our belongings in early November, leaving the cold and the snow and our friends behind for six months. Having the constant connection through e-mail and the cell phone makes being apart from our loved ones quite tolerable.

Making new friends was not really difficult—that's one of the many blessings of being in the fellowship. But I did still feel the dissatisfaction that had troubled me for so long. I think I had felt certain that more sun, a change of pace and location, and freedom from stress would eliminate the depression. That wasn't to be the case. My doctor had predicted as much but respectfully allowed me to consider her suggestion in my own time. Before I reached that conclusion, however, I began another book, the eighth or ninth in the collection of my two dozen to date. I began the book my husband had suggested—an exploration of what other individuals did when their lives underwent the kind of transformation that happens when you leave a career that has been your focal point for a decade or decades. It was certainly a topic I needed to gather wisdom about, and I assumed many others might want the information too. Baby boomers, the biggest single group of future retirees, were soon to come around the bend.

That book's topic became one of the most interesting pursuits I have undertaken as a writer. A number of things made it so. For one thing, my husband took a real interest in it. My life as a writer was very separate from our lives together. He respected and appreciated what I did and thought I did it well; however, recovery self-help books weren't "his thing." This particular book included interviews with many people, and he sat in on most of the interviews. Many of them were done in Minnesota and in Florida. But those done on a trip we made throughout Arkansas really got his attention—and his praise for the way I got people to open up. A bond, perhaps greater than the bond we already had, was the gift we received from making that trip together.

The decidedly incredible element of those interviews, particularly the ones in Arkansas, was that the people who spoke to me didn't know me when I contacted them. They simply trusted that a voice on the phone requesting the opportunity to speak with them about their lives meant no harm. Being told that I was gathering information for a book that I hoped would be helpful to others as they made transitions through life provided the appeal. No one said no. No one. Praise be to God. *Keepers of the Wisdom* was born.

I will always remember the people I met while writing that book, and their words have taken root in my mind. Every time I read one of the daily meditations from *Keepers,* I remember once again exactly where Joe and I sat while in the presence of the person being interviewed. Each one offered me something very specific and special. Each was an artist in her or his own way, and all of them had very "holy" ways of looking at their lives and the world around them.

The truly amazing thing was that they ranged in age from their early seventies into their nineties, and none of them had quit doing what they really loved to do. They had had careers of many kinds but had found their real bliss in other activities as the years progressed. And they were fulfilled, thrilled to awaken every day. And they lived, with the exception of one woman, with the knowledge that God had been a part of their journeys. I learned so much from these wise men and women.

And yet at the time, my own journey was still troubled by a shadowy darkness far too often. As had been the case while still working for Hazelden, if I turned to writing, threw myself into the process of letting *God speak through me,* I felt safe and whole. That's how I continued to survive, until that warm summer day that the antidepressant I so reluctantly tried took effect.

It's with some concern that I have been sharing the part of my journey that includes reliance on medication. I would never want to be considered a role model for others when it comes to this solution for depression. As I have said quite emphatically, I resisted this suggestion by my physician for more than a few years because I had been swayed by the voices in "the rooms" that said drugs of any kind meant you had forfeited your sobriety date.

How glad I am that saner minds finally prevailed. I am at peace. And what's even better, I can and do write with the same, or greater, passion than ever before. God willing this will continue to be true until the day I die.

I don't know that I'll always be on medication; however, my physician and psychiatrist have indicated the probability is great that I will be. Chronic depression seldom heals itself. I have come to terms with that. And I don't deny to others that I have turned to medication for the treatment I need. If they choose to judge me, so be it. I want to maintain a sense of peaceful balance in my life, and this is what I need to do to accomplish that.

ॐ

YOUR TIME TO WRITE: Time for a change of pace. Your opportunity to write is calling now.

- *What brings you the most satisfaction?*

- *Who do you know who seems propelled by an inner bliss?*

- *Why not ask that person or people where their passion came from?*

- *What would you most like to try in your life that you have put on hold for now? Why? What do you need to do to "take it off the shelf"?*

BIRTHING BOOKS

Earlier I had shared some stories about my failed pregnancies. There were five in all, with an ectopic on either end of the series. Losing all of those pregnancies never really bothered me emotionally. Or at least I don't think so. Maybe being an elementary school teacher for eight years compensated for the babies I couldn't have. But I have often wondered whether my childhood intention to never have babies played a role. My mother reminded me well into my thirties that I had always announced to the adults in the family that "I was going to be a working lady, not a mother." After the third grade, I requested that I stop receiving dolls for Christmas. I had already moved on. I do believe our intentions can become the reality in our lives. Many spiritual "gurus" seem to agree.

I had never considered that my "birthing" experience would entail the production of books, but I do think each one of us is called to contribute to this life we share in specific ways. My call has been to write books, most definitely. I laughingly tell others in the workshops I lead that I have given birth twenty-four times to date. The book you are reading right now is number twenty-five. I think God's decision to make me a writer rather than a mother was very wise. This activity has given me ample opportunity to practice, again and again, the principles that are so necessary to my peace of mind. If I had attained the level of balance and contentment I seek, I'd be done writing on these topics. My search continues, as does my writing.

One of the old-timers at an Al-Anon meeting I regularly attend says, "I go to AA so I can live without alcohol. I go to Al-Anon so I can live with people." I'm still a work in progress when it comes to living with people, but I'm committed to practicing the principles that undergird our fellowship.

I've mentioned many times that I'm a writer, but I need to be clear with you that every word in every book came through me, to you, in the same instant that I "heard it."

Nearly like an out-of-body experience, writing happens to me. I sit up and listen and write and am amazed. Twenty-five times I have been amazed. I hope to be amazed at least ten or fifteen more times. After all, I'm only seventy-one!

Going back and forth between Naples and Minneapolis provides its own kind of rhythm, one that I like. It feels as though I'm blessed many times over with friends, good meetings, good weather, and the desire to keep writing, all in the presence of hovering angels in both locations and all spots in between. The work I do can be done comfortably from any location and that's "a God thing" for sure.

There was a time in my life when the work I did didn't feel comfortable anywhere. Experiencing the miracle of surrendering has changed all of that. The miracle of medication has played its part too. Being pushed to the breaking point, as was true for me, has its silver lining if we open the doors that seem to beckon to us.

A READY-MADE FAMILY

Since coming to Naples twenty years ago, we've experienced some major surprises. For one, a son who Joe fathered more than forty years ago surfaced. Joe and the birth mother had agreed to let the boy be adopted without their interference and after reaching adulthood, if the child wanted to find them, they would be open to it. Indeed, it happened. Seventeen years ago, shortly before Christmas, a note arrived from the birth mother announcing that their son had made contact with her and that he wanted to have contact with Joe too.

I opened the card assuming it was a Christmas greeting from a friend to both of us. I read the note and passed it on to Joe, saying, "This will change your f——g life." He was stunned into silence—a rarity for him. He got on the phone, called the birth mother, and got his son's number. They talked for hours, and Joe made plans to fly to Minneapolis that weekend.

From the beginning of our relationship, I had known about the possibility of this happening. I had secretly hoped it would occur, but many years had passed with no contact. And, as so often happens, when we finally "move on," God says, "The time is right." They had a sweet encounter that proved to be the start of a life-changing experience for Joe, and ultimately for me too. One of the sweetest parts of gaining a "ready-made" family was the three-and-a-half year old grandson.

I didn't get to meet the son, his wife, or the child until spring, when we headed back to Minnesota for our annual six-month stay. One of the first dates we made was to gather as a family over dinner. It was a delightful experience to meet the three of them. My new grandson was darling. Polite. Bright. Inquisitive. A blue-eyed blond. I was so excited for the rest of the family to meet him. His gentleness touched my heart immediately. The following week, Joe introduced his newfound family to the extended Casey family, which includes Joe's mother, seven sisters, their spouses, and many nieces and nephews.

Joe and I planned a picnic. The entire family came, all very excited to meet the "new additions," and it was a typically chaotic gathering. Joe's family is nothing if not animated, fun, and loud—all seven sisters clamoring for attention at the same time. Jordan sat quietly by my side while the older nieces and nephews raced around us throwing balls, cursing at one another, and turning hoses on guests. I had grown accustomed to this behavior, but it wasn't pleasant. And no one scolded. In spite of it all, when my grandson left, he walked quietly to my side and said, in a small voice, "Thank you for inviting me to the lovely party." No doubt he had been prompted, but the contrast was glaring—and so appreciated.

A journey that was rife with unexpected pleasures, for me in particular, had begun. Having a step-son, daughter-in-law, and grandson—a ready-made family—filled my heart to overflowing. A second grandson soon came along. Even though I had never envisioned a family in my life, I trusted the process. By now I knew that God opened doors that were marked with my name. I also believed that "my contracts" with others had been earmarked in another time.

For the next few years our lives mirrored those of the more typical families in America. We vacationed together, had weekends at a cabin, went to Disney resorts. Dinners together gave us many chances to really establish a family life. There were glitches on occasion, however. That's typical of all families, and ours experienced growing pains. Over time, the growing pains escalated.

For more than a decade we made the best of things. One blessing, and there is always one within any experience, is the relationship that we forged with Jordan. He's now twenty-one years old and studying in Spain. A remarkable young man who, under my supervision, wrote a book at age ten. Let me share the story. It's a great one. When we return, you'll get all the details.

YOUR TIME TO WRITE: This is a great stopping place. I hope you think so too.

- *Did anyone come into your life unexpectedly? If so, how did that change your journey? Is that person still present? In the same or in a different capacity?*

- *Explore those details and how they added to the experience of your life.*

- *When you look back on that experience, is there anything about it you wish had been different?*

- *What has been its lasting effect, if any? How do you think your presence changed him or her?*

- *If we believe, as I do, that every experience is a stepping stone to the next phase of our life, what phase was that for you?*

- *What phase do you see yourself in now?*

JORDAN'S STORY

Jordan was intrigued by my being a writer. He loved to write too and proudly shared some of his poetry with us. His imagery impressed both Joe and me. By this time, I had written twelve or fifteen books, one of them for young girls, titled *Girls Only!* He excitedly called me one day while I was in Naples and said that a classmate had brought that particular book for show-and-tell. When he told the class that his grandmother had written it, they scoffed. His next request was dear to my heart: "Would you come for show-and-tell when you get home from Florida?" He wanted to prove to them that his grandmother was the real writer.

Our return was later than usual that winter. The last week of classes were in session, but Jordan's teacher allowed me to come, bringing all of my books in tow. I spoke to them about writing and the joy it brought me. I encouraged them to write, even if they thought they didn't know how. One boy asked me if I was going to write a book for boys like the one for girls. I explained that since I wasn't a boy, that would be very hard for me to do. But this little boy planted a seed. After going to Jordan's school that day, I asked him if he might like to write one for boys similar to the one I had written for girls. He didn't warm up to the idea right away, but I would ask him on occasion if he had given it any consideration.

About a year passed when I was at his house one afternoon. He was hanging out with some of his friends and they remembered me from the show-and-tell. One boy asked if I had written a book for boys yet. I replied that I thought Jordan should write it. Many voices chimed in, quickly agreeing. I asked Jordan later that evening if he might want to take a stab at it. He seemed reluctant but interested at the same time. I told him I'd send him a copy of the girl's book for him to look at. I suggested he read the subject index carefully for clues about the topics he might write about.

Surprisingly he called a few days later and said he'd like to try it if I'd help. I agreed to help and told him the sales could create a college fund for him. For the next year, Jordan wrote and I read, even sitting together on occasion at the family dining room table. He used the subject index as a guide for his own topics and then wrote short essays that would appeal to a boy's mind and heart. It was a wonderful little book: *A Boy's Book of Daily Thoughts* by Jordan Storeby. It's still available online and through Hazelden. Like most books, it didn't become a best seller, but it's a feather in his cap and showed him the power of perseverance.

The real blessing for me, and I think for Jordan too, was that we developed a trusting relationship, one that has survived even though the ties with the rest of the family are frayed. Being able to help him go to Spain to study is only one of the gifts I have received from the work I have been led to do. His kind heart will pay it forward when the time comes. I know it.

GUIDANCE FOR GIRLS

My own desire to have written a book for girls, two books for girls, in fact, grew out of my commitment to help others avoid some of the pitfalls that I had fallen into. Because of my overwhelming insecurities as a school girl and teenager, insecurities I've already detailed for you, I wanted to offer some helpful guidance to the younger generation. As an adult, I knew that my clinging to others, my incessant doubting that I was liked when young, made my decisions for me, decisions that were far from healthy. My first drink at age thirteen was only one of my poor choices. Stealing from my first place of employment at age twelve, a pattern I repeated in high school at another job, was setting a pattern that might have claimed me for life. Fortunately, God had another plan.

I hadn't been raised to do what I did, but then I hadn't been given the comforting guidance I needed either. I had received a lot of criticism but not a lot of "good job!" When in doubt about a direction, we choose for ourselves, and the immature, as yet undeveloped frontal lobe of the brain understandably fails to make the good choices. I read a number of years ago that the decision-making lobe of the brain isn't actually fully developed until our midtwenties. That gave me a sense of relief. Unfortunately, I continued to make many very poor decisions even after my decision-making lobe was fully developed, owing to the dis-ease of alcoholism. When that's part of the equation, all bets are off.

I wanted to help girls avoid the pitfalls I experienced growing up and to know early in life that they didn't have to get sidetracked. So I wrote *Be Who You Want to Be* and *Girl to Girl*. And yet by the time I had written those two books, I had become fully cognizant that the sidetracking I had done was an important part of my journey and perhaps would be for my readers too. It's true that wherever we are is where we need to be, whether side track, fast track, or alley. I spent time on all three, and my final destination, for now, couldn't be better. And yet I wanted the young reader to know that regardless of what she was experiencing, she could find comfort in the certainty that a Higher Power is waiting to be asked for help, that the hovering angels are present even though unseen, that other people have gone through the same thing, and that I for one was trying to reach her with a few words of courage and hope. Regardless of age, we need both to keep moving forward.

WRITING AS DIRECTED

The books I have written since *Each Day a New Beginning* cover the gamut of topics that might be of interest to men and women on a spiritual path. Book number two, *The Promise of a New Day,* relied on the principles of the Twelve Steps without referring to any program. It had been my feeling from the time I had gotten sober that everyone in the entire world would be better off, more content and peaceful, if they lived according to the principles that were guiding the lives of all of us in Twelve Step programs. My second book was the solution, I felt.

The Third Step of AA is the focus of *In God's Care.* Loving ourselves and others with greater intensity is the intention of *Worthy of Love.* And *If Only I Could Quit* is a book for treating nicotine addiction—an addiction I chose to get free from during the first few months of my sobriety. It was a rather mystical experience that I'd like to share: I had been ill for a few days and had missed many meetings. My women's AA group came to my apartment, as was typical of us, to put on a meeting. It was December 20, just seven months after my last drink. One woman, Rita, shared that she'd like to give her family the gift of her becoming a non-smoker for Christmas. She said she had tried many times to quit but always, within a week or two, was unsuccessful. I had just that day read John Powell's small book, *He Touched Me,* in which he shared how he had quit smoking. I began to tell her his story. Powell said he changed his personal identity. Instead of thinking of himself as a smoker who had quit, he began to consider himself a nonsmoker at every turn, specifically all those times he would have "lit up" in the past. It became natural. His mind changed. How he saw himself changed. How he responded to others changed too.

After telling Rita of John Powell's story, I put out my Pall Mall Gold and never lit another cigarette, even though I had become a solid, two-pack-a-day smoker. I had not even considered quitting until that moment. I loved smoking in the same way I had loved to drink. Until the moment I stopped drinking, and then stopped smoking, the thought to quit had not crossed my mind. And since those two days, the thought to begin either again doesn't weigh heavily on my mind. I believe it was self-hypnosis that helped me become a nonsmoker. I simply never wanted to smoke again. I can't say that my emotions didn't scream for a hit of nicotine during the first couple of weeks or that I was calm and kind throughout my withdrawal, but the desire to smoke evaporated. Rita also quit using this method.

The decision to write a book to help others make the same choice to quit that Rita and I made was easy. Gathering the stories of how a few dozen others did it was enlightening and engaging. That was the first book I wrote for which I needed to interview others. I realized in the process of that book that interviewing was a special way to encounter others, and that I was actually good at it. Being an attentive, careful listener is an art, I think. I don't know why I have the gift to do it, but I'm glad that's one of the gifts I have been blessed with. We each need a witness. Perhaps feeling as though I wasn't being "witnessed" as a young girl and even as a young adult woman made me ever more committed to doing for others what I had missed out on.

Following the smoking book, I did another book for women: *A Woman's Spirit.* To write it, I was inspired to contact many of the women who had written to me after reading *Each Day a New Beginning.* The correspondence I had received after the publication of that book was phenomenal. I had had no inkling that others felt as I did. It wasn't that I didn't share at meetings or that I didn't talk to my sponsor about some of the things that bothered me. I just played my cards close to my chest, telling only some things because I wanted to control the perception others had of me. Being completely vulnerable was still out of the question.

I wrote to the women asking them to share a small thought, a quote of sorts, that I could use as the theme for a meditative essay. I asked them for permission to use their names. Not one woman declined. Sharing their words, coupled with mine, felt like an honest example of sisterhood. It also demonstrated to me, and hopefully to them, that we need each other one and all, that our journeys are intertwined and intentional, and that the contract to meet *in this way* was decided long ago.

A Course in Miracles, a spiritual program of study that I became a student of in the early 1980s, gave rise to a daily meditation book focusing on the principles of "the Course," titled *Daily Meditations for Practicing the Course.* I wrote it in 1995 at Hazelden's request because so many people had begun to look for help with the material. This course of study has been a mainstay for me since I first opened the text in 1982. It dovetails beautifully with the Twelve Step philosophy that has guided my life since 1974. To have these three spiritual pathways, AA, Al-Anon, and "the Course," sustain me on this journey is undoubtedly a God-given blessing, one that I cherish every moment of the day. There are no accidents. Remember that. What I have been given, where I have been brought, whom I have been introduced to have all been part of the "assignment." The same is true for you. Never doubt that.

The rest of my books followed in due order, one every twelve to eighteen months. I wrote the first five books longhand, and I was afraid the spell would be broken when I turned to the computer to write. God showed up anyway. I know now that God always shows up if we make a space for Him.

The next few books, though along the same spiritual lines, looked dramatically different. I didn't set out to create a contrasting format. The format simply developed organically from the book's intention. That's the real beauty of being inner directed when it comes to an activity like writing. The subject matter doesn't look to me for direction. It pulls me along, much like my dissertation pulled me along so many years ago. At that time, my advisor Dr. Sibley asked me on numerous occasions for a copy of my outline. At long last I had to admit I didn't have one. I dared to tell him I was "writing as directed." He smiled. He actually understood. He said that was a first, but he was okay with it. That has been my process for everything I've ever written since starting graduate school. I can't guarantee others that writing in this fashion will work. Each one of us has to find our own way.

YOUR TIME TO WRITE: This is no doubt a good place to take a break. You have been reading enough from me. Now it's time for you to dig deep into yourself again.

- *Which of your accomplishments do you prize the most?*

- *Have you experienced anything like my husband and I did with children returning to your life?*

- *Do you have grandchildren? If you do, what's the most significant thing you have learned from watching them?*

- *What is the one thing (or two things) you hope you have passed on to them?*

- *If you could relive any experience regarding children or grandchildren, what might that be? How might that "do-over" affect your life and theirs?*

- *If you have a particular skill, describe it. How has it been a blessing? If you think you don't have one, think again. We all do! Ask a friend what she thinks yours is.*

- *What has brought you the most joy, recently, as it pertains to family?*

LESSON-LADEN RELATIONSHIPS

My recent books have focused quite specifically on relationships—those at home, at work, in the back yards of the communities we live in—and how to make those relationships better, particularly more peaceful and nurturing. This is no doubt owing to my own need, as the years slip by, to live a less chaotic, more comforting life. It's also owing to my spiritual commitment to doing my part to make this world we share with more than six billion others less tumultuous. I believe, and I know I'm not alone in this belief, that what we think manifests sometime, some place. If the thoughts I am harboring are hateful toward others, I am hurting those people as well as people I may never get a chance to know. Conversely, I feel it's my work to share kind, thoughtful messages with you for the good that might be expressed throughout the universe. It's my hope that you are inspired to do the same.

Fearless Relationships was my first book to take this subject in hand. Relationships had been my bane for years. From childhood on, I craved them, squeezed the life out of them, cried over them—and went looking for a new one every time one ended. This had been my history until recovery began. It would have continued to be my history had not Kris and Eileen steered me away from relationships when I got into AA. But I was still capable of complicating them when I was "allowed" to get into one. Remember the hideous story about Joe's mosaic and my file cabinets? And years later I can still complicate my primary relationship because of my need to control what's not mine to control. Although I no longer look to my husband Joe or anyone else for my feelings of self-worth, I do have control issues and the subject matter in *Fearless Relationships* called to me.

Telling others what has worked for me, much the way we do in Twelve Step meetings, is how my books seem to evolve. God, working through me, guides others. And in the process, I am reminded too of how peaceful recovery works. I've come to see my role as the intermediary between God and the reader. I am willing to write pages and pages of what *comes to me*. It's as simple as that.

I wrote the book *Change Your Mind and Your Life Will Follow* over summer months, seven very long days every week of the summer, while making the best of our living space on Prior Lake in Minnesota. We had bought an old "tear-down" cabin and then postponed the demolition. My very capable husband Joe did some work to make it livable for the summer months. I sat at a make-do desk and worked on "changing my own mind" as the words tumbled forth. It was one of the easiest books I have ever written. I loved the message and the ease with which it flowed. I knew it was a winner. The e-mails and letters I have received since its publication confirm that in spades.

The fact that relationships were always so painful for me has paid off. I have been comforted by every book I have written, and others have been helped too. We are always directed toward activities that have a role to play in the larger picture of our lives. I used to doubt the veracity of this idea, but no more. There was a reason for the turmoil I experienced. And now I have made good use of it. Turmoil visits all of us. Turning toward it, embracing it for the lessons it offers, is what the hovering angels help us to do. It's their intention to see us through.

I suspect that relationships will continue to be the primary focus for my work as a writer and workshop leader, and that pleases me greatly. I'm comfortable with an audience. I know that anyone who comes *has been called.*

I also know that what they hear will be orchestrated by their Higher Power and has virtually nothing to do with me. That relieves me of any angst I might have about the gathering. My job is to love the people who gather, not to look for love. I'm not in charge of anything except showing up. God is in charge of the rest.

I heard a great story that speaks to this dilemma from John Powell a few decades ago when he offered a seminar in Minneapolis. By this time, Powell had written twenty or more books and led probably thousands of seminars. After he walked to the front of the room, he shared a story that was stunning and so dear. He said that for years he had been terrified of speaking before an audience even though that was what the Franciscans had assigned him to do. He always prayed about it, but the fear wouldn't leave. Finally he spoke to his superior about it, and his superior replied, "John, your problem is that you want your audience to love you. Your job is to love them." From that moment forth, he was no longer afraid. I have remembered those words, and I let them guide my thoughts too. The result is no less than miraculous.

I think all healing happens in relationships and only in relationships. We may think we are "healed," but as soon as we get into a relationship, we are off and running, trailing the many character defects that are still there. All of the old behaviors were just lying dormant. Our dis-ease escalates in isolation. Our healing occurs when we allow others to see us as we are and accept us anyway. Others are helped by our humility and honesty. My journey, your journey requires encounters with others for us to heal. It's that simple. Furthermore, it has been my experience that the relationships that are the most difficult are the most significant and lesson-laden. I have walked away on occasion or been frightened away, but the lessons waited for me. So did the hovering angels.

The following point bears repeating: I feel like a lucky woman to have been chosen as a carrier of this disease, of both of these diseases. I'm sure I was born codependent and alcoholism was my chosen solution. That is, until it worked no more. Then the rooms of Twelve Step recovery became the solution, and they will not quit working as long as I don't quit taking a seat in the rooms where others beckon me in. It's quite exciting to know that I will always have a place to call home, that I will always have a group of friends who love me even though they probably don't know my last name, that I will always have a set of beliefs to guide me when I can't think of a single reason to be kind or comforting or available to others.

When I look back on my life, I find it interesting that a woman who felt so little peace for so many years in her family of origin is in the "business" of *selling* peaceful ideas to others. This proves three things to me: (1) God has a sense of humor, (2) He is always preparing us for what is yet to come, and (3) He will get us to fulfill His plan for our lives by hook or by crook. And to think I fretted in the beginning of my journey when I tried to decipher what God's will for me was. All along He had the perfect plan, which included the perfect solution. And I am fulfilling it joyfully to the best of my ability. How about you? I think the time is right for you to dig a little.

ॐ

YOUR TIME TO WRITE: Healing ourselves is what this journey is about. Are you progressing?

- *What has helped you the most with the healing you have needed to do?*

- *How would you describe your relationships? What has made some better than others?*

- *Do you see yourself repeating some of the old behaviors in new relationships? What do you do when that happens?*

- *What do you see as the most common theme in your relationships? How does this information inform your behavior?*

- *Are you cognizant of how certain behaviors still entrap you? What's your "plan of attack"?*

- *Today, my life feels like a dream come true. Does yours? If not, how might you make it so?*

The Next Teacher

My relationships, in spite of all the writing, coupled with all of the workshops, the meetings, and the sponsees, are far from perfect. I am a work in progress, as anyone who knows me will agree. But that's the blessing of having this kind of dis-ease. We get the rest of our lives to heal it. And it may well be that all we can ever do is arrest it. That's okay too. The tools for arresting it are easily applied, one day at a time, one encounter at a time, one moment at a time.

I remember with clarity the slogans that were hanging from the walls of the first Al-Anon meeting I attended in 1974. I could not, for the life of me, understand what they meant. Oh sure, I could understand the words, just not the subtle meaning behind the words. In fact, I turned my nose up at them, certain that someone as "bright as myself" would not need to be guided by ideas so simple. My progress on this journey may well have been a bit speedier had I looked at those slogans more carefully and with a greater openness.

When I review my life, looking particularly at the significant relationships I know I was meant to have, I'd give myself at best a B-minus grade overall. In my first significant relationship, I clung like a drowning rat, terrified of letting my high-school boyfriend Steve go lest I be left behind for good. Claiming him as "my booty" didn't bode well for us. He became the first of many who abandoned me. My security was tied to *having and being "a partner,"* not tied to a relationship with a God of my understanding. I wouldn't even have known how that idea could fit in the overall plan for my life.

I'm not even deserving of a passing grade in my first marriage, but I did show up every day for twelve years. My attendance was good. Unfortunately, my deportment wasn't. It's true that I was doing the best I could based on the information I had at the time. I wasn't tuned in to the kinds of ideas that inform my thoughts and actions on a daily basis now. I hadn't even been introduced to these ideas through books or role models. The result is that I wasn't a loving partner. I didn't even desire to be a loving partner. I was intent on wishing him harm because of my hurt feelings. When we can't love one person, we fail to fully love anyone really. That's what I have come to believe.

The same principle applies when we consider forgiveness. If we are holding a judgment against one person, we are blocking ourselves from the peace of mind that we deserve. Unforgiveness keeps us separate from our brothers and sisters, and separation leads to the dis-ease that can hold us hostage for a day or a lifetime. I was imprisoned until I began to seriously incorporate the principles of the Twelve Step programs that were and are my lifelines. Adding the core beliefs found in *A Course in Miracles* has been like adding a layer of whipped cream on an already delicious chocolate cake. I need never falter when deciding what to do or say. The principles for right action are readily available.

I've learned enough while on this journey to not shame myself for the many mistakes I made earlier in life. Although on occasion I do have remorse about not being able to show up in a very loving way in my family of origin or my first marriage, I know I was simply held hostage by my own sense of inadequacy, which drove me to actions that were hurtful to others. *Hurt people hurt people,* as they say. I've seen this played out in the lives of others too, including my father.

As I've said, in one way or another on many occasions, our relationships are the training ground for the healing we have been born to experience. They are not accidental or happenstance, but quite intentional. Every one of them. And the awareness of that has become a true blessing. I don't have to sort out anymore *Why him or her?* I don't have to ask the proverbial question *Why me?* I don't need to ponder something that feels unfair. What happened with Steve and John and Brad and particular family members with whom emotional or physical boundaries were crossed all added to the tapestry of color that has become my life. And everything that happened *there and then* has added "a bit of color commentary" to those relationship issues that have surfaced with Joe during these last three decades. Nothing in our life's experiences can be considered a throwaway, never to be heard from again. Everything is recycled. Everything.

When I reflect on relationships, even the seemingly minor ones, I'm reminded of the book *The Five People You Meet in Heaven* by Mitch Albom. It was an intriguing look at an idea that resonated with me. Our "meetings" with others, no matter how fleeting or supposedly inconsequential, may have contributed down the line to a significant turn of events that we'll be able to "see" when we get to the other side. I do believe I "missed getting hit by a lot of buses" on my journey. The number of "buses" that missed me because someone got my attention for a moment, changing the time of my departure at the last minute, was exactly as it needed to be.

I am excited about seeing my five, or my twenty-five people, when I get to heaven. Although I think I know who some of them are, I also know there are dozens of others who have escaped my recall and dozens more who haven't even registered on my radar screen. I love the set of beliefs that guide me now. I don't worry about the future. Or the present. Nor do I fret over the past. I know I met the experiences with as much grace as I was capable of at the time.

Whenever I sort through the many relationships that triggered anxiety in me, I realize they were similar in "content." I was generally in a reactive mode to someone else's attempt to control how I thought or acted. My dad, my first husband, my boss when I was in high school, and my boss while I worked at Hazelden were all strong men, and I was and continue to be a strong woman. My fear propelled me to respond to their fear. Fear is always the initiator of anyone's need to control or attack. The great lesson in this is that we simply can't ever control anyone else. And until we learn that, we will continue to "meet" those people who seem to tax our serenity. Now when someone comes into my life and gets under my skin, I know it's because I want to change him or her. And sooner than in years past, I recognize the person as simply the next teacher on my educational path.

YOUR TIME TO WRITE: Perhaps it's time for you to look within again.

- *Who have obviously been "your teachers"?*

- *Whom do you think you might meet in Heaven?*

- *Who are the people you think you affected most along your journey and theirs?*

- *What's the most interesting thing you have to say about your relationships?*

- *Are there some relationships that still make no sense to you?*

- *If you agree that relationships are our vehicles for healing, what specific relationships do you think you have been healing in this life?*

- *What is your spiritual "profile"?*

- *Are you content with it? If not, how do you want to change it?*

What It's Like Now

ॐ

FORGIVENESS AS THE WAY HOME

L IFE IS NOTHING if it's not interesting. I certainly didn't
knowingly chart this journey for myself. And yet I believe I absolutely had a sizable part in its creation. I am
also convinced that my journey has been perfect up to
now and will remain so. Every day upon waking, I know
my feet are on stable ground doing exactly what God has
intended. I feel certain the same is true for you too, and
if you are having trouble believing that, let me hold that
belief for you.

It's been important for me to admit to, even embrace,
all the darkness I was attracted to. It got my attention far
more often than the "kittens and the daisies" that called
to many of my friends. Did I think I wasn't deserving of
the kinder, softer experiences when I was young? Or did
I march to the beat of a different drummer because that
route had been predetermined? Even to this day I occasionally hedge my bets about what I believe in regard to
predetermination, God's loving will, and my own role in
the script I have been living. I do know, however, that the

events of the past can't be changed. The present is where my blessings lie, and the future has no hold on me yet.

Being a child in a raging, dysfunctional family in which alcohol was ever-present—although my parents were not engulfed in the daily disease of alcoholism—prepared me for the many steps I took between my first drink at age thirteen and the full-blown codependent alcoholic I became by age twenty-one. My confusion and my pain from so many experiences along the way have served as lifelines to others who have looked to me as a sponsor in the days since I chose sobriety. Keeping in mind that all of our experiences will serve us for good at some time or place is comforting. It has assured me that the same will continue to be true. Therefore, I truly do not worry about any of today's activities or any of those that might appear on the "calendar" for tomorrow. They have been *agreed to,* and I have been fully prepared.

The abuse at the hands of a distant relative, the humiliation over the behavior of my dad in front of friends, the incessant tension in our house, and the constant fear of abandonment—all left their mark on who I was determined to become. My "grooming" was intense, often painful, but also strengthening, and I wouldn't trade any of it if that meant giving up the life I get to live now.

I want to remember, and I suggest you remember too, that not all memories of life before recovery are bad. Many are good. Some are very good, in fact. Even though the acrimony in my family made my self-assurance spotty at best, we had some great times as a family that deserve savoring: playing board games, going to ball games, eating at the Frozen Custard stand, and swimming, boating, and fishing at a lake cottage in the summer. My experiences with my grandparents were wonderful and always highly anticipated. My success as a student, a young writer, and young public speaker are still cherished. When I factor in what I have come to believe about the preparation we are always being given for the next "events on our schedule," I relish the depth and the breadth of the experiences I have had, whether good or bad. In one way or another, they have all contributed to the content of the many books I have been compelled to write. Nothing in our lives is for naught. We are where we are supposed to be. We have always been where we were supposed to be.

NEGATIVES AND POSITIVES

I've intentionally left out many details of my life and over-looked others. This memoir is not meant to be definitive. Seventy-one years of detail would fill many volumes, and that's not the point of this guided memoir. It is intended to help you look at the positive and negative memories of your life, strengthening your understanding that from another perspective it is all good. Just being open to the idea that our experiences are part of an individualized learning curve that "wears our name" is freedom for many of us. Life doesn't happen to us. We aren't victims. We're architects.

I went from being an anxiety-ridden child to a promiscuous young adult to an adulterous woman who ran the streets in search of drugs, alcohol, and men. Along the way I married, divorced, got sober, earned an advanced degree, remarried, and became a best-selling author. Looking at life in shorthand doesn't establish how finely tuned the many facets of the journey have been, but they do fit together like the pieces of a puzzle. Not one experience was extraneous. Perhaps you're thinking that swiping Joe's mosaic to the ground could have been avoided. Maybe so, but the lesson we each learned as a result of those few moments of insanity was vital to the rest of our journey. I can surely point to other stories that weren't "pretty," but in each case I became wiser. I know the same is true for you, whatever your experiences have been.

We can take any experience or grouping of details and ask, *Was this really necessary?* And the answer will always be the same. Yes, because each one of us is a grouping of lines on the big drawing board of life. If any of the lines are forgotten, the picture lacks the detail that continues to clarify the emerging image.

We can't undo the past, but we can promise to never repeat it. Regarding my first husband, I wish I had understood the gravity of his alcoholism and insecurities. I know in my heart that his behavior resulted from a mind that suffered. He was not a bad person, and yet I punished him with my thoughts and my actions. I wish I could have a "redo" with some of the experiences we had, but I have been given a chance, in marriage number two, to avoid mistakes I made earlier. I think that's what the curriculum is about. We get the assignment; we fail at it; the lesson comes again.

Through these nearly thirty-four years with Joe and the thirty-six years of my recovery journey, I have experienced phenomenal changes. Most I could never have predicted nor even wanted had God spoken directly in my ear and said, "Karen, this is what I have planned for you." I believe I would have pleaded with him to not "take away the drink." Or the drugs. Or the cigarettes. Or the many failed, unhealthy relationships. Had I heard Him say, "You will be an alcoholic, but you will recover. You will write many books and do workshops around the country and the world," I'd have no doubt resisted. At least I would have resisted the idea that I was an alcoholic. And yet here I am—happier than any woman has a right to be.

LISTING CHANGES

Before I bring this memoir to a close, I want to acknowledge at least a smattering of the many changes in my life and my belief system. You can see these in the list on the next page. I want you to begin making a list of all of the ways you have changed too. Another reason for writing down our lists is so that we can see how hard we have worked. The effort that goes into becoming the men and women we'd rather be is astounding. We need to honor that effort.

What Is Important to Me Now

1. I do not spend my time correcting what I perceive as the "errors" others might be making. (I'm still a work in progress when it comes to my husband, though.)

2. I practice (though I'm not yet perfect) saying nothing rather than offering unsolicited advice.

3. I offer the hand of kindness or a ready smile to everyone I meet in a workshop or even on the street when I am walking. I believe the day's experience can be changed for every person who receives one of my smiles.

4. I believe in the value of service work, and I commit to it readily. A simple yes is all that's required.

5. I never say no to a request to be a sponsor, but I do sometimes say I can only be a temporary one.

6. I do not tell others how to live.

7. I refrain from getting into conflicts. Instead, I use the phrase "You might be right" and let the dust settle.

8. I no longer doubt the timing of the experiences I have. I know that all things are working on God's time frame.

9. I fervently believe that I am meeting the people I am meant to meet and having the experiences I am supposed to have.

10. I no longer fret about the future. I know that it has been taken care of.

11. I do believe I will never have an experience of any kind that God has not already prepared me for.

12. I never doubt "my calling," and I know God will help me fulfill it at every turn.

It was not all that many years ago that I would have received a failing grade on all of the points I listed. I had no spiritual or moral compass and was afraid all of the time about the present and the future. And the past was a horror story. All of that has changed because of one single decision: I got into Twelve Step recovery, first for my dependence on others and next for my dependence on drugs and alcohol. Discovering there was a solution to handle both problems gave me an entirely new perspective. Hope was born in me and nothing about my life has stayed the same.

Of course, I have had *emotional slips* when it comes to letting the others in my life live their journey without my interference. At least once a day I say something that might have been better left unsaid. But I have not been afraid to leave my house. I have not been suicidal. I have not doubted that God is present or that hovering angels are close at hand. In other words, I have made immeasurable progress and will keep doing so.

It's with such relief that I'm able to sit here today and feel content with my life, my work, my relationships, and my intentions for what might come next.

ॐ

YOUR TIME TO WRITE: Before ending this journey we have been making together, I'd like to give you the opportunity to do a bit of reflecting too.

- *When you ponder where you are, as opposed to where you were, what comes first to mind?*

- *What are those specific changes you have made that have blessed you and your family members alike?*

- *What's the most unexpected change you have made?*

- *What one experience encouraged the most changes?*

- *If you could relive your life, what would be the first thing you would change?*

- *Of all the changes you have made, which one seems to be the easiest to stay committed to?*

- *Which change needs your constant commitment to stay on course?*

- *Of which change are you most proud?*

- *What two or three changes are you still hoping to make in your lifetime?*

- *How have you discerned what changes you needed to make?*

Let's look again at the details of our life as we close this activity. It's my hope that it has been as rich and rewarding for you as it has been for me.

THEN AND NOW

When I got sober, I figured it meant a life without alcohol. Period. How wrong I was. How shortsighted I was. The blessings that have been added to my life since walking the path of recovery are so numerous that I can't possibly name them all. To begin with, the friends I've made and what they have added to my life are beyond description—every one of them could walk me through any situation that seemed to be more than I could handle alone. My husband Joe, who is a phenomenal learning partner, is the icing on the cake. I never imagined marrying a man who was to become my best friend, a helping mate like no other, and a constant source of amusement. He never fails to be my teacher, and some days I'm a pretty good student.

If I were to hold up a picture of how I looked shortly before sobriety and then a few months into sobriety, would the ordinary person be able to detect any difference? I'm guessing yes, even though the main difference was within me. Even after a few short months I had far fewer lines on my forehead, I was told, and my hair had a sheen to it that had been missing. I had begun to regain a few pounds too. The lack of good nutrition and the reliance on amphetamines had kept my weight very low for many years. I was way too thin.

Perhaps one of the main differences was my easy laughter. For many years, I think I had lost the willingness to laugh. There didn't seem to be much to laugh about. No relationship partner was "controllable," providing the security

I craved, which meant I had no freedom from anxiety any day of my adult life. I didn't know what to expect from day to day, year after year. I felt as though I were in the waiting room of life, not knowing what I wanted to have happen. I was only certain that it hadn't happened so far and that I didn't have much hope it ever would.

In my early thirties, I wrote a poem titled "Waiting." It was a sophomoric lament about the multiplicity of ways I had waited around for others, primarily men, to pay me some attention. Of course they didn't show any interest in changing in any of the ways that would have allowed us to have a productive relationship. It was a bit embarrassing to read when I came across it a few years ago, but it was a fair assessment of my state of mind when I wrote it. It had been my state of mind for many years, and it remained my state of mind into the first few years of my recovery. I was a willing hostage to any man who paid even a little attention. Waiting for the crumbs was a sick, shameless habit. Letting those few crumbs of attention define me was all I knew how to do at the time.

It has been humbling to write this memoir, to dredge up my dark past in such a public way for unsuspecting eyes. But if I have learned anything on this journey to health and wholeness, it's that secrets keep us stuck and sick. I want to be healed. I am assuming the same is true for you or you wouldn't have embarked on this journey with me. Much of what I have shared is information my family members wouldn't even want to read. It's my hope that you, the reader, will take it in stride. We share this spiritual path. We know the importance of "digging deep." We know the downside of holding back. So it's all out there. And I'm glad.

It's hard for me to bring this memoir to a close because it's been a labor of pure love. Looking at my journey and "observing" the details God laid out for me has been affirming, to say the least. If I ever doubted that God had my back throughout my life, that doubt was dispelled during this process. If for no other reason, that's why everyone should write a memoir. We do need to cherish the evidence of God's presence throughout our lives. It's far too easy to overlook all the times we were saved from ourselves.

A FIVE-YEAR INTENTION

The final area for us to address is intentions for the next few years of our lives. It's perhaps best to at first limit ourselves to the next five years. Within that segment, we might make a discovery that will take us in a wholly new direction for the following five years. When I think of the next few years, at my age, I don't anticipate any big changes. I love my life, my work, my friends, and my willingness to share what God sends to me. I have made it clear to the universe, however, that I am "available" to carry my message wherever God sees fit for me to carry it.

Making an intention known, in fact, affirming it daily, whether verbally or visually, can help to set it in stone. When I was new in sobriety, my friends and I made "picture boards" that made it perfectly clear where we hoped our lives would go and what we hoped our lives would include. Our assignment was to look at the board periodically throughout the day and carry in our minds the pictures we had created on the board, not unlike the visualizing exercise I used when I was preparing for my oral exam. My picture board had details on it that did come to fruition within a couple of years. The intention I am focused on presently is as follows:

I want to be of maximal service, to men and women everywhere, through my books and workshops, both nationally and internationally. Just show me how and open the doors, God.

I'm not sure what gives the power to an intention. Perhaps it's simply that we have surrendered to God what is God's to orchestrate. I do know that intentions open our minds. They allow us to see more clearly who we want to be, where we want to go, and how to get there. And I know they open doors. I feel confident that with all that has come to pass in my short seventy-one years, there is much more good just on the other side of the next door I'll reach—and then the door after that.

The doors that open before you have been inspired by your intentions. It's time now for you to consider what those intentions should be. They belong to you—no one else. Your past has prepared you for any direction that calls. Remember that. That's the only reason our past is of value, in fact—as preparation. The experiences are gone. Only the education remains.

༈

YOUR TIME TO WRITE: Let's quietly meditate awhile before we begin this last exercise. It's the final step on this courageous undertaking.

- *Have you ever made a picture board to draw what you long for? If yes, do you remember what you included? Did what you longed for transpire?*

- *Did that experience change the direction of your life? (It often does.)*

- *If you were to create a list of intentions, or even one intention right now for this next year, what speaks to your heart?*

- *Do you feel prepared to attempt it? Would you believe that you are most definitely prepared for it, or is it something that would not have even occurred to you?*

Our minds can't fathom the impossible. That may seem far-fetched, but it's absolutely true. If you can imagine creating or attaining something, you can accomplish it. The details may have to be engineered, but the finish line is only a brief "moment" away.

I love this kind of belief system, don't you? It takes the angst and anxiety out of the day-to-day experience.

Bless You

And now on to living one intentional day at a time. With our hearts and minds full of hope, let's cherish each day as the gift it is—and doubly cherish each person as he or she approaches us. Each wants to hear what we have to say. We need to hear their responses too. "Our dance" has been previously orchestrated.

That you and I have had this opportunity to weave our stories as one has been a blessing to me. If this is the first time you've encountered me, thank you for trusting this process. If you have been a follower for a while, I can't adequately express my gratitude for your continuing support. Indeed, we are lifelines for each other, lifelines that I hope will never fray.

As one of my dearest friends says with frequency, "Bless your heart for being here." Until we meet again, remember, God and the hovering angels have your back and all is well. This I promise to be true.

ABOUT THE AUTHOR

Karen Casey, Ph.D., is the author of many books devoted to the enhancement of one's personal and spiritual journey. Her first book, *Each Day a New Beginning: Daily Meditations for Women,* has sold more than three million copies. She has published twenty-four additional books and offers workshops and lectures throughout the United States and the world. Her website www.womens-spirituality.com features a blog, her event schedule, and information about new books as they are published.

Hazelden, a national nonprofit organization founded in 1949, helps people reclaim their lives from the disease of addiction. Built on decades of knowledge and experience, Hazelden offers a comprehensive approach to addiction that addresses the full range of patient, family, and professional needs, including treatment and continuing care for youth and adults, research, higher learning, public education and advocacy, and publishing.

A life of recovery is lived "one day at a time." Hazelden publications, both educational and inspirational, support and strengthen lifelong recovery. In 1954, Hazelden published *Twenty-Four Hours a Day,* the first daily meditation book for recovering alcoholics, and Hazelden continues to publish works to inspire and guide individuals in treatment and recovery, and their loved ones. Professionals who work to prevent and treat addiction also turn to Hazelden for evidence-based curricula, informational materials, and videos for use in schools, treatment programs, and correctional programs.

Through published works, Hazelden extends the reach of hope, encouragement, help, and support to individuals, families, and communities affected by addiction and related issues.

For questions about Hazelden publications,
please call 800-328-9000
or visit us online at hazelden.org/bookstore.